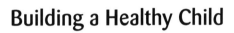

Building a Healthy Child

Building a Healthy Child

Food Introduction Nutritional Program—
A Parent's Guide to Foundational
Childhood Nutrition for Lifelong Health

MELINA ROBERTS, N.D.

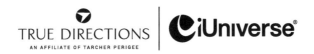

TRUE DIRECTIONS
AN AFFILIATE OF TARCHER PERIGEE

iUniverse®

BUILDING A HEALTHY CHILD
FOOD INTRODUCTION NUTRITIONAL PROGRAM—
A PARENT'S GUIDE TO FOUNDATIONAL CHILDHOOD
NUTRITION FOR LIFELONG HEALTH

iUniverse books may be ordered through booksellers or by contacting:

iUniverse
1663 Liberty Drive
Bloomington, IN 47403
www.iuniverse.com
1-800-Authors (1-800-288-4677)

Because of the dynamic nature of the Internet, any web addresses or links contained in this book may have changed since publication and may no longer be valid. The views expressed in this work are solely those of the author and do not necessarily reflect the views of the publisher, and the publisher hereby disclaims any responsibility for them.

Any people depicted in stock imagery provided by Thinkstock are models, and such images are being used for illustrative purposes only.
Certain stock imagery © Thinkstock.

ISBN: 978-1-4917-8362-7 (sc)
ISBN: 978-1-4917-8364-1 (hc)
ISBN: 978-1-4917-8363-4 (e)

Library of Congress Control Number: 2015919144

Print information available on the last page.

iUniverse rev. date: 2/12/2016

To my amazing child, Addison, who was my inspiration for writing this. I am truly blessed to have you in my life.

Contents

Acknowledgments

Thank you to my wonderful colleagues and friends for reading my manuscript and giving me guidance and the encouragement to publish this project.

Thank you to my parents and brother for their continued support and always believing in me.

Thank you to my husband and daughter for allowing me the time and space to be able to write this book.

Thank you to my patients for continuously teaching and inspiring me.

Introduction

I am a mother and licensed naturopathic doctor (ND). As an ND, I combine the wisdom of nature and modern science to identify and remove barriers to good health and help facilitate the body's innate ability to heal itself. I designed this nutritional program because this is what I was looking for when I had my child. When I was a child I suffered greatly with allergies and eczema, and later I wanted to know what I needed to do to prevent allergies and eczema in my child, as well as to promote long-term health. I also see a lot of patients with chronic diseases in my practice and have come to understand that healing the digestive tract is the key to achieving better health. I wanted to figure out a way to build a healthy digestive tract right from the beginning so that we can prevent common childhood illnesses, as well as chronic diseases. As I started to research and better understand how the systems of the body develop and mature, and as I learned more about our microbiome, the ecosystem of microbes that live in our digestive tract, I began to realize that the way most books tell parents to introduce foods can actually be detrimental to children's health, as these foods do not contribute to proper development of the organs or the proper development of this microbiome. I could find no book that gave parents the appropriate guidance on introducing foods with these concepts in mind.

That was how I came to write this book. This is the kind of information I know parents are hungry for. I have come across many parents who want to prevent food allergies, food sensitivities, and digestive discomfort and illnesses in their little ones but are unsure what to do. As a naturopathic doctor, I have come to realize that the only way to prevent disease in future generations is to build a solid foundation of health in our children.

Most parents want the best for their children and want to give them a head start in life. The one task of parenting that would have the most significant effect on performance is also the area that is the most neglected. We as a society greatly neglect proper nutrition for our children and have been misguided for many years. We feed our children poor nutrition, introduce certain foods too early, put a strong emphasis on poor-quality foods, and then somehow expect our children to develop into healthy, intelligent, successful leaders.

This nutritional program is based on years of research and clinical experience with thousands of patients. The program I share in this book is guided by my knowledge of the development of the human body and the understanding that different organs and systems of each child's body develop at different times. All our organs begin development in utero, they continue to develop once outside the womb, and they reach full maturation at different stages of development. Because of these staggered rates in development, I recommend specific nutrition at particular times in your child's life. We need to follow the body's development and give the growing child the proper nutrition at each stage of growth to ensure proper development. My nutritional plan promotes proper child development and will help you and your family prevent childhood illnesses such as allergies, asthma, and eczema, as well as chronic degenerative diseases (such as cancer and diabetes) later in life. This is a program for true preventive medicine.

When it comes to language development, we don't expect our children to come out of the womb with a full vocabulary and comprehension of the language we speak. We understand that this brain-development skill will take time to evolve, and there is a natural progression that occurs over an extended period of time.

We need to look at the development of our digestive tracts and introduction of nutrition in the same fashion. We cannot expect our children's organs to function and have the same capabilities as fully developed and matured adult organs. Our little ones' organs do not have the same capabilities as mature adults'; their organs are still maturing and growing. It is important to follow the natural evolution of the body to get the maximum benefits of health.

Another key component of this plan is that it takes into consideration the fact that the quality of our food is completely different from our ancestors' food. In fact, most of the food on the market today is different than it was even fifty years ago. The business of agriculture and the promise of higher yields, increased food production, cheaper prices, and greater availability has changed our natural foods to chemical-laden and genetically modified sources. Genetically modified organisms (GMOs) have had their DNA specifically changed by genetic engineering techniques, making the foods more resistant to herbicides or viruses to allow for less damage to crops, potentially leading to higher yields, but the problem has been that these changes were made without the understanding of the possible long-term effects on human health.

The program presented in this book is a clinically significant, well-researched plan that understands the toll these alterations to our foods can take on our health. It was created with the intention of raising children in the twenty-first century among these challenges.

Most experts believe the prevalence of food allergy is rising along with a general rise in the incidence of allergic conditions. Asthma is one of the most common causes of emergency-room visits in Canada. In Canada, 12 percent of children and 8 percent of adults have asthma.[1] In the United States, 8.3 percent of children and 7 percent of adults have asthma.[2] My nutritional program has the potential to greatly improve these staggering statistics and eliminate food allergies and associated conditions if foods are introduced according to the natural evolution of the body.

Three Reasons This Nutritional Program Is Vitally Important

- Digestive health is the key to long-term health.
- The foundation of our digestive health is formed by age three.
- Our organs mature at different rates, and we need to introduce foods to support proper maturation.

---

[1] "Statistics Canada, Canadian Health Survey, 2010," last modified Feb. 11, 2013, http://www.statcan.gc.ca/pub/82-625-x/2011001/article/11458-eng.html.
[2] National Health Interview Survey, National Center for Health Statistics, Centers for Disease Control and Prevention, United States, 2013.

Four key components to understanding the human body make this nutritional program uniquely different from any other food introduction nutritional program:

- Infants have hyperpermeable digestive tracts. This means their digestive tracts absorb materials much more easily than those of adults; therefore, we have to be very cautious what we put into their digestive tracts.
- Our pancreas does not reach full maturation until approximately age two, so we should not be introducing grains until age two.
- We have acquired our own unique foundation of microbes in our digestive tracts by age three, and this will affect our future health.
- Our bodies are hardwired to process real food, so we need to feed our children real, nutrient-dense foods.

This program is designed for parents who

- understand that nutrition is central to good health;
- want to make health a priority for their child and family; and
- want to do everything they can to build a solid foundation for the future and encourage proper growth and development.

It takes time, effort, and diligence to raise a healthy child, but it's worth it.

CHAPTER 1
First Foods

The way most parents are told to introduce foods (i.e., introducing cereals as a first solid food) is the worst way to do it and can set our children up for health issues in the future. Cereals are essentially manmade foods that are refined, processed, and stripped of nutrients, which means they are not "real" food. We can easily prevent this by introducing "real" foods in line with how our organs mature and how our bodies are able to effectively break down and absorb the foods they are given.

The Developing Digestive Tract

When we are born, our digestive tracts are hyperpermeable. (Hyperpermeable means that anything, including food particles that haven't completely been broken down and come into the digestive tract, can easily move through the walls of the digestive tract into the bloodstream.) This means we have to be cautious of what we put into our children's delicate, immature digestive tracts.

The digestive tract is hyperpermeable for a reason: an infant receives its innate (or nonspecific) immune system, as well as all the nutrients, hormones, enzymes, and healthy bacteria they need in order to grow and develop, from the mother's breast milk.

The immune system and digestive tract are immature in a newborn, and the process for preventing food reactions has not been fully activated. For this delicate, immature digestive tract, the only source of nutrition should be breast milk, the perfect food for an infant. There is nothing equivalent to it. Breast milk decreases infections, allergies, and autoimmune reactions in infants. The World Health Organization (WHO), a specialized agency of the United Nations that was established in 1948, recommends exclusively breastfeeding for the first six months to achieve optimal growth, development, and health.[3] Exclusive breastfeeding means offering no other food or drink, not even water, for the first six months.

I recommend exclusive breastfeeding for at least six months and breastfeeding for at least one year. The WHO recommends breastfeeding until two years of age (or even beyond). We should all be aware that the worldwide average of children being weaned from breast milk is 4.2 years old.[4] Unfortunately, in our Western culture, breastfeeding a toddler is considered abnormal, but the longer you can breastfeed, the more beneficial it is for your child's health.

Introducing anything other than breast milk can be damaging to the infant and set up the potential for health issues in the future. Introducing cow dairy–based formula into the infant's hyperpermeable digestive tract causes the proteins to easily move into the bloodstream, whereby the body sees these proteins from the formula as foreign bodies and activates an immune response within an immune system that is extremely immature. This is extremely challenging for a developing infant. The energy within the body goes toward handling the foreign bodies and the activated immune system, which leaves less energy for proper growth and development.

The results can be disastrous in some children, as shown by the statistics from a study published in *Diabetes Care*.[5] The study evaluated the incidence of type 1 diabetes from birth to seventeen years old in Colorado youth and found that type 1 diabetes in children younger than age four showed the fastest rate of increase seen, with an increase in the incidence by 3.5 percent per year. Children who were exposed to cow's milk before four months of age had a 50–60 percent increased risk of developing type

---

[3] World Health Organization, http://www.who.int/topics/breastfeeding/en/.

[4] World Health Organization, http://www.who.int/topics/breastfeeding/en/.

[5] K. Vehik, RF Hamman, D. Lezotte et al., "Increasing Incidence of Type 1 Diabetes in 0- to 17-Year-Old Colorado Youth," *Diabetes Care* 30, no. 3 (March 2007): 503–9.

1 diabetes.[6] We can prevent this debilitating chronic disease by changing the way we introduce foods.

Benefits of Breastfeeding to the Infant

Breast milk contains all the nutrients an infant needs. It is easily digested and assimilated. The breast milk contains immune cells and antibodies that support a healthy immune system and inhibit the growth of harmful bacteria and viruses in babies' developing bodies. Breast milk promotes the development of a healthy digestive tract, as it contains bifidus factor, which promotes the growth of Lactobacillus bifidus in the infant gut and helps build the foundation of healthy microflora.[7] Breast milk contains hormones and growth factors that help in the maturation of the mucous membranes of the digestive tract.[8] Breast milk contains essential fatty acids, which are necessary for optimal brain and nervous system development. Breast milk contains antibodies known as immunoglobulins A, M, and G (immunoglobulins identify and bind to infectious agents and kill these invading microorganisms).

The first few days after delivery of your baby, the breasts secrete a clear fluid called colostrum. This is the perfect food for your baby. It is easily digested, loaded with immunoglobulins, including immunoglobulin A (IgA), which stimulates the development of the infant's immune system. Colostrum has higher levels of IgA and white blood cells, which protect newborns against infections. Colostrum also helps newborns' digestive tracts grow and develop.

A newborn has a specific immunity from the mother that lasts for the first three months. Breastfeeding provides the infant with additional maternal antibodies and immune-enhancing factors. A baby's immune system is not able to produce antibodies necessary to fight infections. Babies acquire this ability over the first few years of life as they are exposed to viruses and bacteria.

---

[6] HC Gerstein, "Cow's Milk Exposure and Type I Diabetes Mellitus: A Critical Overview of the Clinical Literature," *Diabetes Care* 17 (1994):13–19.

[7] S. Pathak, U. Palan, *Immunology: Essential and Fundamental*, 2nd ed. (New Hampshire: Science Publishers Inc, 2005), 215.

[8] Ibid.

What is interesting is that the nursing mother makes antibodies in response to microorganisms threatening the baby. When the baby is invaded by an offending virus or bacteria, the infectious agent is passed from the baby to the mother as the baby nurses, and then the mother produces matching immunoglobulin and sends the protective agents back to the baby through the breast milk.[9] This is a brilliant, innate protective system that cannot be duplicated.

Lucas et al.[10] published research in *Lancet* that assessed whether nutrition in early life has a long-term influence on neurodevelopment. Three hundred children who were born prematurely were evaluated. Those who were breastfed in the early weeks of life had higher developmental skills at eighteen months. Those same children previously breastfed from age seven and a half to eight had an 8.3 point higher IQ than those who were formula fed.

A study done in 2010 and published in the *Journal of Allergy Clinical Immunology*[11] found that children who were breastfed exclusively for more than four months had a reduced risk of asthma in comparison to children who were breastfed fewer than four months. The breastfed children also had better overall lung function.

Benefits of Breastfeeding for the Mother

Breastfeeding also has benefits for the mother:

- It is a wonderful way to bond with your baby. There is a huge emotional connection that happens between the mother and baby through breastfeeding. This early bonding is important for the baby's developmental and emotional health.

---

[9] Ibid.

[10] A. Lucas, R. Morley, TJ Cole, G. Lister, C. Leeson-Payne, "Breast Milk and Subsequent Intelligence Quotient (IQ) in Children Born Preterm," *Lancet* 339, no. 8788 (Feb. 1, 1992): 261–4.

[11] I. Kull, E. Melen, J. Alm et al., "Breastfeeding in Relation to Asthma, Lung Function, and Sensitization in Young Schoolchildren," *Journal of Allergy and Clinical Immunology* 125, no. 5 (May 2010): 1013–9.

- During breastfeeding the hormone oxytocin is released, which helps the uterus contract and return to normal size more quickly.
- Typically, weight loss is faster in mothers who breastfeed, because you burn more calories when breastfeeding.
- Studies have shown that breastfeeding reduces your risk of breast,[12] uterine, and ovarian cancers,[13] decreases rates of depression,[14] and lowers the risks of developing osteoporosis.[15]

Mother's Diet during Breastfeeding

It is important for moms to avoid certain foods when breastfeeding. All the foods that she eats will be transmitted to the breast milk and can cause sensitivity or an allergic reaction in the infant.

Breastfeeding mothers should avoid

- alcoholic beverages (cause of fetal alcohol syndrome)
- cow's dairy (causes inflammation)
- wheat (causes inflammation)
- corn (majority is GMO)
- tomatoes (highly acidic food)
- white refined sugar (causes inflammation)

Breastfeeding mothers should limit their consumption of

- eggs (limit to once every four days because of potential sensitivity to albumin in egg whites),
- pork (limit to once a month because of contributing to possible autoimmune problems),

---

[12] JL Kelsey, MD Gammon, EM John, "Reproductive Factors and Breast Cancer," *Epidemiological Reviews* 15, no. 1 (1993): 36–47.

[13] RB Ness et al., "Factors Related to Inflammation of the Ovarian Epithelium and Risk of Ovarian Cancer," *Epidemiology* 11, no. 2 (Mar. 2000): 111–17.

[14] JJ Henderson, SF Evans et al., "Impact of Postnatal Depression on Breastfeeding Duration," *Birth* 30, no. 3 (Sep 2003): 175–80.

[15] RG Cumming, RJ Klineberg, "Breastfeeding and Other Reproductive Factors and the Risk of Hip Fractures in Elderly Women," *International Journal of Epidemiology* 22, no. 4 (1993): 684–91.

- soy (limit to once a week because of the majority being GMO), and
- coffee (limit to one cup per day because of the caffeine depleting the adrenal function).

If your breastfed baby experiences any of the following symptoms, this may suggest the baby is trying to eliminate a substance that does not agree with his or her body. Symptoms can often be treated by eliminating these allergenic foods from the mother's diet.

- rashes
- wheezing
- eczema
- colic
- spitting up
- vomiting
- painful gas
- constipation
- diarrhea

Mother's Supplements during Breastfeeding

Breastfeeding is an unequaled way to make sure your baby is receiving optimal nutrition and is a good start toward building a healthy immune system and for emotional nurturing. While you are breastfeeding, it is important to maintain a healthy diet to support the demands of your growing baby.

Women who are breastfeeding should continue to take the high-quality supplements taken during pregnancy, including B complex, a multivitamin, calcium-magnesium, essential fatty acids (EFAs), and probiotics. EFAs are extremely important in the early development of the baby, especially their neurological systems, and levels in the breast milk are correlated with the mother's intake.[16]

In addition to daily supplements and to aid in recovering from labor

---

[16] JM Krasevec et al., "Maternal and Infant Essential Fatty Acid Status in Havana Cuba," *American Journal Clinical Nutrition* 76, no. 4 (Oct. 2002): 834–44.

and delivery, mothers who are breastfeeding may consider alfalfa, a great healing herb that is a rich source of vitamins A, C, E, and K, as well as calcium, potassium, phosphorus, iron, and trace minerals.

Some problems associated with breastfeeding can be effectively addressed with natural supplements. Here is a list of common challenges associated with breastfeeding and some strategies to help you overcome them:

Milk Production

Red raspberry leaf, alfalfa, fenugreek seeds, and blessed thistle have been used traditionally either individually or steeped together as a tea to increase milk production. Red raspberry leaf tea also helps restore the reproductive system after childbirth.

Mastitis

Inflammation of the breast, or mastitis, can be treated by applying cool, green cabbage leaves to the affected breasts or by boiling dandelion root in water, cooling, and making a compress. If an infection is the cause of inflammation, it may be beneficial to take a garlic supplement, a potent natural antibiotic, as well as echinacea to boost the immune system and fight the infection.

Sore Nipples

Dry, cracked nipples are a common problem with breastfeeding. They can be treated by applying chamomile cream or coconut oil as an antiseptic ointment that is safe for mom and baby. Squaw vine, applied topically as a salve, can also be used to treat nipple soreness.

Breast tenderness

Some breast tenderness is caused by water retention. As parsley is a diuretic, parsley extract can be taken as a supplement to help flush excess water from the body. Caution must be taken when consuming parsley while breastfeeding, as consuming large amounts may reduce milk production.

Weaning

When it comes time to reduce milk production in preparation for weaning, applying the crushed fresh flowers of jasmine to the breasts has been shown to inhibit lactation. Mint and/or sage teas have also been shown to help reduce milk production.

The Problem with Formula

Formula was originally designed for orphans who, due to unfortunate circumstances, could not receive the benefits of breast milk. Now formula is advertised as an equivalent replacement to breast milk, but this is entirely inaccurate.

Cow's dairy formula is very different from breast milk. Cow's milk is low in iron and copper and vitamins A, C, and E. Cow's dairy is a hyperallergenic food. Introducing this food before twenty-four months can lead to an allergy issue.

Most formulas are cow dairy based. Cow's dairy is made up of casein, a large protein that is difficult to properly digest, even for adults with mature digestive tracts. When this protein is introduced too early, it passes through the baby's delicate, underdeveloped digestive tract into the bloodstream, where the immature immune system has to deal with it. Often the immune system will tag the cow protein as a foreign protein. This ends up being a challenge for the infant's system. Any challenges to the baby's body can affect proper growth and development.

Soy-based formulas can also cause similar challenges, as soy is a difficult protein to break down, and most soy and soy products sold on the North American market are genetically modified. A better alternative to cow dairy–based or soy-based formula would be goat or sheep formula. These are not easily accessible, and you may need to make them yourself, but the advantage is that the goat or sheep caseins are smaller proteins, larger than breast milk but smaller than cow's milk, and are easier to metabolize.

The common practice of giving cow's dairy to infants is undoubtedly a major contributing factor to higher incidences of food sensitivities, digestive disturbances, and chronic diseases.

Formula-fed babies have higher incidences of rashes, wheezing, colic, and vomiting. The intestinal lining may be so severely damaged by early cow's milk consumption that a person will remain sensitive throughout his or her life and have numerous food and environmental sensitivities. This is the common source of immune deficiencies and chronic diseases later in life, including asthma, eczema, and diabetes.

Formula Replacement

At this time there is no beneficial formula on the North American commercial market. The commercial formulas are either made from cow's dairy protein or soy protein. I understand that some mothers are unable to breastfeed for a variety of reasons or will not have enough milk to meet their growing babies' needs. I would suggest making homemade formulas. See chapter 8 for homemade baby formula recipes.

Supplements for Newborns

For newborns I recommend live, specifically formulated probiotics. They can be administered by putting the powder on your finger and having the baby suck the powder. Typically, if this is done at least three feedings a day, it should be enough of a dose to have a positive influence on building a healthy gut flora foundation. This is extremely important for the developing digestive tract and has been shown to prevent ear infections, eczema, asthma, colic, constipation, and diarrhea in babies.

CHAPTER 2
Problem Foods

The Problem with Cow's Dairy

Our bodies cannot effectively break down cow's milk. It sits in the digestive tract and causes inflammation, which is a self-protective mechanism to remove harmful substances from the body and begin the healing process. Cows are routinely given hormones and antibiotics to make them grow faster, bigger, and stronger, and these substances make their way into the milk that is consumed by humans. Specifically, recombinant bovine growth hormone (rBGH), a genetically engineered artificial hormone, is injected into dairy cows to make them produce more milk, and unfortunately this chemical ends up in the cow's milk. The problem is there has been little to no research done on the long-term effects of these hormones and antibiotics on human health.

The commercialization of cow's milk has made it a lot different than it was even fifty years ago. Back then cow's milk was freshly squeezed and delivered to your door on the same day from a local farm, where you knew exactly where the milk was coming from, what the farmers were feeding the cow, and how the cow was being treated.

The dairy industry is very different now; it is a big business industry. Cows are given hormones to make them produce more milk than normal and antibiotics to try to ward off infections and fatten them up. The milk is pooled together from a number of different cows and different farms. It is then heated in a process called pasteurization, which kills off any bacteria in the milk, but it also kills off any healthy bacteria from the milk and denatures (ruins) beneficial enzymes. This leaves the milk with a lot fewer beneficial substances and a lot more chemicals than it had fifty years ago. Due to the homogenization and pasteurization process, milk no longer has beneficial bacteria and enzymes.

The Pottenger cat study[17] showed that cats that were fed pasteurized milk showed skeletal changes, lessened reproductive efficiency, and had respiratory problems, with each subsequent generation worse than the previous. (See more about this study in chapter 3.)

Alternative: Leafy Greens for Calcium

When I tell my patients to avoid cow's dairy, the typical question that follows is, "But where will I get my calcium?" It is true that cow's milk has a high percentage of calcium, but what does that cow eat in order to have that high calcium content? Green grass. The most easily absorbed, bioavailable form of calcium is from green leafy vegetables. Consuming two to three servings per day will provide your daily calcium requirements.

Another question I get is, "Can I get enough calcium from vegetables? I'm worried about getting osteoporosis."

Let's talk about how the body really functions and the truth behind the osteoporosis/calcium/cow's dairy connection. Cow's dairy is an acidic food, so every time you intake cow's dairy you are causing your body to become more acidic. Your blood is very sensitive to this acid-base balance and needs to keep the pH within a very narrow range. When you start consuming acidic foods, such as cow's dairy, wheat, sugar, or alcohol, your blood works to buffer this acidity by pulling minerals, including calcium, out of the bone to bring the blood into a healthy pH range. I do not dispute the calcium content in milk, but if you can understand how the body biochemically functions, then you can see that cow's dairy actually contributes to osteoporosis. We see this statistically, as the Western world has the highest incidence of osteoporosis in the world,[18] as well as the highest consumption of cow's dairy. Green leafy vegetables are

---

[17] F. Pottenger, *Pottenger's Cats: A Study in Nutrition* (California: The Price-Pottenger Nutrition Foundation Inc. 2009).

[18] DK Dhanwal, C. Cooper, EM Dennison, "Geographic Variation in Osteoporotic Hip Fracture Incidence: The Growing Importance of Asian Influences in Coming Decades," *Journal of Osteoporosis,* Article ID 757102 (2010).

alkaline (the opposite of acidic) foods, and the bioavailability of calcium is quite high; therefore, you can get enough calcium from eating your vegetables, which also helps ward off osteoporosis.

Alternative: Goat's Milk

Goat's milk contains a smaller, more easily metabolized version of the protein casein. Goat's milk contains higher amounts of essential fatty acids than cow's milk, and these types of fat are easier to digest. Agglutinin, which causes fat globulins to cluster, is part of cow's milk but not part of goat's milk. All goat's milk on the commercial market in North America is pasteurized, but most are antibiotic-free and often not given extra hormones, which is commonly part of a cow's diet. I recommend goat's milk as an alternative to cow's milk. I suggest introducing organic goat's milk to your baby around one year of age.

The Problem with Grains

In terms of the maturation of the human organs, the pancreas does not reach full maturation until about twenty-five months. Therefore, we cannot effectively break down grains until around two years of age. This is why I recommend that we not introduce grains to children until this time.

Seven thousand years ago in ancient Egypt there were northern Egyptians and southern Egyptians who were essentially genetically similar. The northerners began farming and agriculture and lived off a diet that mainly consisted of grains. The southerners were hunter-gatherers, having a traditional diet and living off game meat, fish, and vegetables. When you look at the mommies, the northerners' mouths were filled with rotten teeth and metal (thus the beginnings of dentistry), while the southerners had nearly perfect teeth.[19]

Dr. Weston Price, a dentist and author of *Nutrition and Physical Degeneration*,[20] studied primitive populations to better understand tooth

---

[19] R. J. Forshaw, "Dental Health and Disease in Ancient Egypt," *British Dental Journal* (2009): 421–4 doi:10.1038/sj.bdj.2009.309.

[20] W. Price, *Nutrition and Physical Degeneration* 6th ed. (California: the Price-Pottenger Nutrition Foundation Inc. 2000).

decay. He found that the populations that ate a diet dependent on their environment had flawless teeth, well-proportioned bodies, perfect skin, shining hair, clear eyes, and pleasant dispositions. Whole, real, natural foods were the key to their robust health, and it affected the next generation.

Dr. Loren Cordain, author of *The Paleo Diet,*[21] uncovered similar findings. The archaeological records of ancient humans with grain-focused diets had ill health, showed high rates of infectious disease, had more childhood mortality, shorter life spans, osteoporosis, rickets, bone-mineral disorders, cavities, and jaws that were too small for their teeth.

The Problem with Wheat

Wheat is made up of a protein called gluten. This is a very large protein that is difficult to effectively break down and metabolize. Since our bodies cannot effectively break it down, it will sit in our digestive tracts and cause inflammation.

Modern wheat is very different from the wheat our ancestors ate a hundred years ago. The proportion of gluten protein in wheat has increased enormously as a result of multiple generations of hybridization. Pure wheat flour has been processed into refined white flour that is stripped of its nutritional value. The wheat was hybridized to have a high gluten content to produce a stronger dough structure and improve baking quality, as well as to supply a high-protein bread. The problem is that the further our food is from its natural form, the more difficult it is for our bodies to recognize and effectively metabolize it. Our food has changed due to economics, not for the best interest of people's immediate or long-term health.

Studies in mice genetically susceptible to type 1 diabetes show that the elimination of wheat gluten reduces the development of diabetes

---

[21] L. Cordain, *The Paleo Diet* (New Jersey: John Wiley and Sons Inc., 2002).

from 64 to 15 percent[22] and prevents intestinal damage characteristic of celiac disease.[23]

Another problem with wheat is the conventional farming practices with the application of the herbicide Roundup (which contains the active ingredient glyphosate), to the wheat crop, which is used to kill off unwanted vegetation. In the 1980s farmers did a preharvest application of the herbicide Roundup to wheat. In the late 1990s many conventional farmers began a practice called "desiccation," whereby they spray the wheat crop with glyphosate just before harvest. When you expose wheat to a toxic chemical like glyphosate, it releases more seed, resulting in a greater yield of crop and an earlier harvest.[24] This leads to glyphosate residues in conventional wheat products.

Glyphosate has been shown to disrupt the balance of gut bacteria; increase the ratio of pathogenic bacteria; damage the villi in the gut; and impair cytochrome P450 enzymes, which play an important detoxification role in the body. It has been connected to chronic diseases that are rooted in gut dysfunction, including celiac disease, gallbladder dysfunction, fatty liver, and pancreatitis.[25] There is an extremely strong correlation between of the use of glyphosate and increases in different diseases, including celiac disease, autism, type 1 diabetes, autoimmune disease, thyroid disease, kidney failure, and cancer.[26]

I recommend introducing wheat at two years of age at the earliest, but never make this food a staple in your child's diet. There are a number of alternate grains to consider, including spelt, barley, rye, oats, quinoa, and kamut. These alternate grains are preferable to introduce after the age of two.

---

[22] DP Funda, A. Kaas, T. Bock et al., "Gluten-Free Diet Prevents Diabetes in NOD Mice," *Diabetes Metabolism Research and Reviews* 15 (1999): 323–7.

[23] F. Maurano, G. Mazzarella, D. Luongo et al., "Small Intestinal Enteropathy in Non-Obese Diabetic Mice Fed a Diet Containing Wheat," *Diabetologia* 48, no. 5 (May 2005): 931–7.

[24] A. Samsel, S. Seneff, "Glyphosate, Pathways to Modern Diseases II: Celiac Sprue and Gluten Intolerance," *Interdisciplinary Toxicology* 6, no. 4 (Dec. 2013): 159–84.

[25] Ibid.

[26] Ibid.

Melina Roberts, N.D.

The Problem with Soy

Approximately thirty years ago a geographic epidemiology research study[27] on soy evaluated the health of Asian populations and observed that they had less breast cancer, prostate cancer, and cardiovascular disease; fewer bone fractures; fewer hot flashes in woman; and lower incidences of age-related brain disease. They questioned why the Asian population was healthier and free of many common diseases seen in the Western world. One conclusion was that the soy in their diet, which was not commonly seen in the Western diet, made a big difference.

So the Western world started to consume soy in all different forms, and in true Western fashion they consumed it in large amounts. With the increased demand came an agriculture business that needed to keep it up. It began to make higher yields in shorter periods of time, and thus came fertilizers and genetically modified sources to aid in meeting this demand. Unfortunately, now in the twenty-first century, most of our soy sources are genetically modified and chemically laden.

The truth is the Asian populations consumed small amounts of fermented soy (like miso, tofu, and tempeh) from non-genetically-modified sources. If you are able to find organic, non-GMO, fermented soy products, these are acceptable to consume in limited quantities.

The Problem with Corn

Corn is a common food sensitivity. We are most familiar with corn in its kernel state, but it is also found in many processed foods. A large percentage of corn on the market today is genetically modified to have increased resistance to insects and pests. The genetic modification to corn includes the *Bacillus thuringiensis* crystal protein gene being transferred (grown) into corn, allowing the corn to produce its own pesticides against insects. These are considered advancements in agriculture that have gone through rigorous testing and been approved by the FDA, but the

---

[27] Barrett JR, "The Science of Soy: What Do We Really Know?" *Environmental Health Perspectives* 114, no. 6 (June 2006): A352–8.

potential risks on short- and long-term human health still remain to be rigorously studied.

Another problem with corn is that pesticide residue from surrounding soil tends to accumulate and become concentrated in the kernel of the corn, making it a high source of toxic pesticides when consumed.

The Problem with Refined White Sugar

Refined white sugar is all over the place: in candy, soda, baked goods, most processed foods, commercial sauces, and salad dressings. It is a hugely problematic substance in our diet. There are numerous reasons we should avoid feeding refined white sugar to our children.

It starts off as a natural plant from sugar cane or sugar beets, and then through heating, mechanical, and chemical processing, all vitamins, minerals, proteins, fats, enzymes, and fiber are removed until only the sugar remains. Sugar is stripped of all nutrients, providing zero nutritional value. Refined white sugar is not a food. It is a pure chemical derived from plant sources.

What is left is a highly refined, isolated, concentrated, chemically manipulated version of a plant source. All the manipulation actually makes it an unnatural product and more of a drug-like substance.

Sugar feeds unhealthy bacteria and fungi in the gut, which leads to an overgrowth of unhealthy bacteria and fungi and an imbalanced microbiome, and since about 80 percent of the immune system is housed in the digestive tract, this leads to a depleted immune system. Sugar destroys the germ-killing ability of white blood cells for up to five hours after ingestion. It decreases the production of antibiotics, which are the proteins that bind and inactivate foreign invaders in the body. It interferes with the transport into cells of vitamin C, a nutrient that plays a vital role in the functioning of the immune system. Sugar causes mineral imbalances, which weaken the immune system.

Sugar rapidly increases blood glucose levels, which stimulate insulin production by the pancreas and make the pancreas work much harder than it needs to. Over time this can lead to a weakened pancreas, insulin resistance, and eventually diabetes.

Sugar is an addictive substance that stimulates the feel-good chemical called dopamine. Most addictive drugs increase dopamine production in the same way sugar does.[28] This demonstrates the chemical addictive component of sugar.

If sugar is consumed and not required in the body, it is stored as fat. The overconsumption of sugar is a contributing factor leading to the overweight and obesity epidemic and all its associated risk factors. The average American child consumes about thirty-four teaspoons of sugar every day. This overconsumption is a growing problem that has led to an epidemic of childhood obesity.

Too much sugar in the blood damages nearly every cell and can cause severe long-term damage to the body, as it is a major inflammatory substance.

Alternatives to White Refined Sugar

Acceptable natural sweeteners include real maple syrup, raw honey, pure stevia, and coconut palm sugar.

---

[28] P. Rada, NM Avena, BG Hoebel, "Daily Binging on Sugar Repeatedly Releases Dopamine in the Accumbens Shell," *Neuroscience* 134, no. 3 (2005): 737–44.

CHAPTER 3
Solid Food Introduction

Why Is Digestive Health Important?

Digestive health is the key to long-term health. We are what we eat! What we eat literally becomes every cell in our body, so what we eat and how our digestive tracts absorb nutrients from the foods we eat dictate the health of our body. The better shape our digestive tracts are in, the better health we are in.

Our digestive tract is a big part of our immune system. It is the barrier that decide what gets into our body and what stays out. If the integrity of the digestive tract is compromised in any way, unwanted substances can make their way into the body.

The other important aspect of our digestive tracts is that about 80 percent of the lymphatic system is housed there. This is the system that drains and cleans up our tissues and moves unwanted substances out of the body. If the lymphatic system gets congested, it can affect the body's ability to clean up tissues and effectively move unwanted substances out. A new discovery recently found lymphatic vessels directly connecting the lymphatic system to the brain.[29] This means that if toxins or chemicals get into the lymphatic system from the digestive tract, the developing central nervous system can be vulnerable to circulating toxins, hence affecting brain development and function. This link makes digestive health even more important for proper immune function and brain health.

---

[29] A. Louveau, I. Smirnov et al., "Structural and Functional Features of Central Nervous Lymphatic Vessels," *Nature* (March 20, 2015); 523: 337–41.

Allergy Prevention

In the Pottenger cat study,[30] cats were given a diet that was not ideal for their digestive tracts, consisting of cooked meat and heated milk. These cats developed all kinds of allergies. They would sneeze, wheeze, scratch, be irritable, nervous, and not purr. If this diet was continued, the second generation had greater incidence of allergies. By the third generation the incidence was almost 100 percent. When the second-generation animals returned to an optimal raw-food diet, their allergic symptoms began to diminish. By the fourth generation some cats showed no evidence of allergies. This study suggests that having an optimal diet can prevent allergies from developing in our offspring.

In a study involving human health,[31] the three main areas for reducing the incidence of allergies were being breastfed exclusively for the first four months; early diet of fruits, vegetables, and healthy fats; and probiotics.

Common Signs of Allergies

The following are all common signs of food allergies or intolerances. These are ways your body is possibly trying to eliminate the allergen. The following symptoms may occur following the introduction of a new food:

Respiratory Tract Symptoms

- runny nose
- sneezing
- wheezing
- stuffy nose
- watery eyes
- recurring ear infections
- persistent cough

---

[30] F. Pottenger. *Pottenger's Cats: A Study in Nutrition* (California: the Price-Pottenger Nutrition Foundation Inc., 2009).

[31] S. Tricon, S. Willers, H. A. Smith et al., "Nutrition and Allergic Disease," *Clinical and Experimental Allergy Reviews* 6 (Aug. 2006): 117–88, doi: 10.1111/j.1365-2222.2006.00114.x.

- congestion
- rattling chest when breathing

Skin Symptoms

- rash
- hives
- swelling in hands and feet
- dry, scaly, itchy skin
- dark circles under the eyes
- puffy eyelids
- lip swelling
- tongue soreness

Intestinal Symptoms

- mucousy diarrhea
- constipation
- bloating
- gassiness
- spitting up with every feeding
- vomiting
- intestinal bleeding
- poor weight gain
- rash or redness around anus
- abdominal discomfort

Solid foods should be delayed as long as possible. The more mature the infant's digestive tract is at the time of solid food introduction, the more likely he or she will be able to tolerate the food. The longer you can wait to introduce foods, the more time you give the digestive tract to fully develop. This reduces the development of allergies, asthma, eczema, and chronic disease.

Infants are not designed for early food introduction. Infants are designed to suck, not chew. An indication of that is that teeth will not appear until around six or seven months of age. Infants do not have good coordination of the tongue or swallowing movements. Infants are born with a tongue-thrust reflex that causes the tongue to automatically protrude outward when any foreign substance is placed in the mouth. This is a mechanism that protects the baby from choking on solids given too early. This tongue-thrust reflex diminishes between four and six months of age.

An infant's small intestines are hyperpermeable, meaning they have higher absorption capabilities in comparison to an adult's. The intestines also have limited digestive capacity due to a lack of development of all the necessary digestive enzymes. Therefore, an infant's digestive tract can absorb incompletely digested (metabolized) proteins that accumulate in the body. The body has no beneficial use for these proteins and starts to create a reaction. The infant's immature immune system may identify these proteins as potentially harmful. This can appear symptomatically as common childhood disorders such as colic, abdominal bloating, gas, constipation, diarrhea, skin rashes, eczema, ear infections, mood swings, irritability, and behavioral problems.

New Solid Foods

New solid foods should be introduced in small quantities in the morning, which is the best time to start so you can see a reaction if it occurs during the day, as opposed to introducing a new food at dinner and then putting the child to bed and potentially having a reaction overnight. If he or she has no adverse reactions, you can increase the amounts. Reactions can include sneezing; runny nose; rash or redness around the mouth, anus, or urethra; a change in stool; a skin reaction; or changes in personality.

Introduce a new food every four days. This gives the body a chance to process the new food and be ready for the next. During those four days the parent/guardian/caregiver watches for any signs or symptoms that the child is exhibiting an allergic reaction or sensitivity.

Ideally, consuming organic, non-genetically-modified foods is preferred in order to reduce the toxic load on the liver. No food is perfectly free of contaminants and toxins, but an effort will have been made to reduce the toxic load when you consume organic, non-GMO foods.

For premature babies, I recommend introducing foods according to their adjusted age based on their due date and not their actual birth age.

Six Months

Begin with hypoallergenic vegetables that are easy to digest. Cooking, pureeing, and/or mashing foods breaks down bonds and makes the foods easier to digest and metabolize. Also, the lack of teeth at this stage makes chewing solid foods a challenge, so sticking to pureed and mashed foods is easier to handle and prevents choking.

Here are some foods to introduce at six months:

- acorn squash
- asparagus
- artichoke
- avocado
- broccoli
- carrots
- cauliflower
- green peas
- sprouts
- squash
- string beans
- sweet potatoes
- yam
- zucchini

Eight Months

Fruits have a higher concentration of natural sugars, so we want to introduce these foods after hypoallergenic vegetables so that the infant has a wider taste spectrum than just sweet foods. Most fruits are more acidic than vegetables, and this is why you want to wait until about eight months to introduce fruits. Cook all fruits, as this makes it easier for an infant's digestive tract to metabolize.

Here are some foods to introduce at eight months:

- apple sauce
- apricots

- bananas
- beets
- blackberries
- blueberries
- cherries
- grapes
- kiwis
- nectarines
- papaya
- peaches
- pears
- plums
- prunes

Ten Months

At this stage you can introduce proteins and some tougher-to-metabolize vegetables.

Here are some good foods to introduce at ten months:

- beef (organic, grass-fed)
- cabbage
- chicken, organic
- egg yolks
- fish, wild (not shellfish)
- lamb, organic
- parsnips
- spinach
- Swiss chard
- turkey, organic

Twelve Months

Many babies are being weaned off breastfeeding at this stage, and this is a good opportunity to introduce goat's milk. Goat's milk has many of the beneficial nutrients that are contained in breast milk; the main protein, casein, is slightly larger than breast milk but small enough that it is easier to digest and metabolize than cow's milk. This is also the time you can introduce more acidic fruits and vegetables.

Here are some good foods to introduce at twelve months:

- goat's milk
- oranges
- pineapples
- tomatoes

Eighteen Months

At this stage you are starting to introduce some easy-to-metabolize complex carbohydrates. This is the time to introduce shellfish, as the digestive tract is more developed and the immune system is more mature, which can ward off immune responses. These can be hyper-allergenic foods, especially if introduced too early.

Here are some examples of carbohydrates and shellfish to introduce at eighteen months:

- beans
- legumes
- nuts
- rice
- seeds
- shellfish
- split pea soup
- quinoa

Twenty-Four Months

Around twenty-four or twenty-five months the pancreas reaches full maturation. Therefore, we are able to properly digest and metabolize grains, so this is the best time to introduce grains. With a better-developed digestive tract, microbiome, and immune system, this is also a good time to introduce the hyper-allergenic foods. Egg whites have a protein in them called albumin that many infants' sensitive digestive tracts react with. Delaying the introduction of eggs can avoid this potential allergy or sensitivity. You can introduce wheat and cow's dairy, but these foods should never be staples in your child's diet. You can make exceptions on special occasions such as birthdays and holidays.

Here are some examples of grains and hyper-allergenic foods to introduce at twenty-four months:

- amaranth
- barley
- buckwheat
- corn
- cow's dairy
- eggs
- millet
- nuts (except peanuts, since peanuts are a hyper-allergenic food and should be avoided until age three)
- oatmeal
- soy
- spelt
- wheat

Three Years Old

In recent years there has been an increase in anaphylactic allergic reactions to peanuts. There are many theories as to why this increase has occurred. I suspect it is related to the genetic modifications that have been done to the peanut and the difficulty for our bodies to recognize this change and properly metabolize this substance. Other contributing factors to this epidemic are that peanuts are prone to harboring molds, since they grow at the same level as mold, most notably the carcinogen aflatoxin.[32] Peanuts also have a tendency to accumulate pesticide residue from surrounding

---

[32] MA Mahmoud, "Detection of Aspergillus Flavus in Stored Peanuts Using Real-Time PCR and the Expression of Aflatoxin Genes in Toxigenic and Atoxigenic A. Flavus Isolates," *Foodborne Pathogens and Disease* 12, no. 4 (April 2015): 289–96.

soil and become concentrated sources of toxic pesticides. This has created a new challenge for the children of the twenty-first century, which results in our needing to delay the introduction of this food as long as possible, to a point when the child's digestive tract and immune system are more developed.

In terms of trying to avoid this serious allergy, the longer you can delay introducing this food, the less chance of having an allergy to this food. This is due to the fact that the longer you wait, the more time you are giving the digestive tract and immune system time to mature.

General Guidelines

Exclusively breastfed for at least six months
Breast milk for at least one year
Avoid grains until two years old
Avoid egg whites until age two
Avoid nuts until age two
Avoid peanuts until age three

Food Introduction Chart

Age	Category	Examples
birth to 6 months	breastfed only	
6 months	hypoallergenic, cooked vegetables	acorn squash, asparagus, artichoke, avocado, broccoli, carrots, cauliflower, green peas, sprouts, squash, string beans, sweet potatoes, yam, zucchini
8 months	cooked fruits	apple sauce, apricots, bananas, beets, blackberries, blueberries, cherries, grapes, kiwis, nectarines, papaya, peaches, pears, plums, prunes

Age	Category	Examples
10 months	proteins; tougher vegetables	beef, cabbage, chicken, egg yolks, fish, lamb, parsnips, spinach, Swiss chard, turkey
12 months	goat's milk; acidic fruits and vegetables	goat's milk, oranges, pineapples, tomatoes
18 months	complex carbohydrates; shellfish	Beans, legumes, nuts, rice, seeds, shellfish, split pea soup, quinoa
24 months	grains; cow's dairy; hyper-allergenic foods	amaranth, barley, buckwheat, corn, cow's dairy, eggs, millet, nuts (except peanuts), oatmeal, soy, spelt, wheat
3 years	peanuts	

CHAPTER 4

Other Considerations When Introducing Solid Foods

Organic Foods

Organic foods are grown without the use of pesticides or synthetic chemical fertilizers. They should not contain genetically modified organisms (GMOs). They contain no artificial food additives or chemical ripeners and are not subjected to food irradiation. Animals are not given antibiotics or growth hormones and are fed foods that are not chemically laden.

Some countries, including Canada, Australia, the European Union, and the United States, have higher standards for being able to claim certain foods are certified organic.

It is difficult for any food in our toxic world to be completely organic, as it's hard to prevent pesticide sprays from nearby nonorganic farms from contaminating the organic farms among them, or the air pollution to not affect our crops, or to have a truly clean water supply that won't contaminate the food supply. So, yes, even with every effort made by great organic farmers, it is difficult to have completely clean foods, but organic foods are cleaner foods that will reduce the intake of toxicity into our bodies. They are better options than nonorganic foods. It is recommended that you feed your little ones organic foods whenever possible. By reducing the toxic load, we allow our bodies to function optimally with little interference to the system's growth and development.

We fed our daughter exclusively organic foods for the first two years of her life. Now at the age of eight, she is not completely on organic foods now, but we do primarily buy organic, non-GMO, locally grown more often and when available.

Melina Roberts, N.D.

GMO Foods

GMOs (genetically modified organisms) have had their DNA specifically changed by genetic engineering techniques. Many of the alterations were done to make the foods more resistant to herbicides or viruses to allow for less damage to crops, potentially leading to higher yields. This sounded appealing to most farmers. The problem has been that these changes were made without the understanding of the possible long-term effects on human health.

These foods are genetically different from their natural origins. Our bodies have been hardwired throughout history to break down foods that are part of nature. When foods are manipulated and changed, our bodies have a challenging time recognizing them, properly breaking them down, and metabolizing them. Biochemically, the body may see these foods as foreign bodies and treat them as toxins, ultimately making the food of no nutritional value. Or the food can be incorporated into our cellular DNA, which has the potential to cause damage as the altered or manipulated DNA should not be part of our cellular structure. The possible implications on our health are unpredictable.

Animal feeding tests have shown worrying health effects. Here's an example: GMO sweet corn contains Bt toxins, designed to protect the plant by rupturing the stomach of an insect that feeds on it. Monsanto (arguably America's forerunning multinational agrochemical and agricultural biotechnology corporation that is responsible for most GM crops around the world and the producer of the toxic glyphosate-laden herbicide Roundup) claims the toxin will break down before it is consumed by us, but when rats were fed the GMO corn, they showed organ failure,[33] and the toxin has been detected in the bodies of pregnant women.[34]

The potential risks of GMO foods on our human health are more

---

[33] J. Spiroux de Vendômois, F. Roullie, D. Cellier, GE Séralini, "A Comparison of the Effects of Three GM Corn Varieties on Mammalian Health," *International Journal of Biological Sciences* 5, no. 7 (2009): 706–26.

[34] Aris A, Leblanc S., "Maternal and Fetal Exposure to Pesticides Associated to Genetically Modified Foods in Eastern Townships of Quebec, Canada," *Reproductive Toxicology* 4 (May 31, 2011): 528–33.

than troubling and challenging to avoid in North America due to the laxity of our labeling laws. If you live in Europe, avoiding GMO foods is easier since laws require labeling. However, in the United States and Canada food manufacturers are not required to label whether their food is genetically modified. This makes it challenging to completely stay away from GMOs. Avoid feeding your children genetically modified foods. We need to demand proper labeling of GMOs so we can make a choice whether to consume them.[35]

Making Your Own Foods

This can be a challenging and time-consuming task, but making your own baby food will have a huge benefit on your child's health. I suggest making big batches and freezing them in ice-cube trays and pulling them out as needed.

Have you ever tasted jarred baby food from the grocery store? It doesn't taste like the actual food it claims to be, as it is processed and filled with preservatives and additives to make it last longer on the shelves. One benefit of making your own baby food is that you can control what goes into your homemade versions. There shouldn't be any preservatives, additives, or sugars when you make your own. This is an economical way to ensure fresh foods that are nutrient dense and free of additives.

Your baby gets a sense of what the actual food tastes like, so when the time comes to move on from pureed or mashed foods and introduce finger foods, he or she will be able to recognize the taste. Children who eat homemade foods are more likely to be good vegetable eaters as they grow up.

Microwaves and Our Health

The first domestic microwave oven came onto the market in the 1950s. It was sold as a quick and easy way to defrost or heat up food. It is now a common household kitchen appliance and is in most homes in the

---

[35] See http://civileats.com/2015/07/20/5-things-to-know-about-the-dark-act/ for more information about the current debate revolving around US labeling laws.

Western world. Unfortunately, no reliable research was done on the effects of microwaved foods on human health prior to the release of this highly used appliance. In 1975 a histological study, published in the *Journal of Food Science,*[36] revealed that when broccoli and carrots were microwaved, there was deformed molecular structures of nutrients to the point of destroying cell walls, in comparison to conventional cooking, where the cell structure remained intact.

When proteins are microwaved, a high percentage of the protein's configuration is altered, and this makes it difficult for our bodies to properly metabolize these foods.

Lubec et al.[37] conducted a study, published in *Lancet* in 1989, on microwave-heated infant milk formulas. It found that a high percentage of proteins' configuration was altered at a molecular level, specifically in the cis-tran formulation, which means the structure of the protein is physically changed because of microwaving. Lubec et al. stated that "the conversion of trans to cis forms could be hazardous because when cis-amino acids are incorporated into peptides and proteins instead of their trans isomers, this can lead to structural, functional, and immunological changes." Therefore, we should not microwave foods for our babies or ourselves.

In 1994 the *Journal of the American College of Nutrition*[38] found that the quantity of proteins changed when infant formula was microwaved, producing molecular changes in the amino-acid components in milk proteins that cause toxicity and compromise the nutritional value of the formula.

When plastic is microwaved, the chemicals from the plastic leaches into the foods, increasing the foods' toxicity. Bisphenol-A-diglycidyl (BADGE) is a cold-cure adhesion used in plastic packaging and many plastic bottles. This is a toxic chemical for human consumption and

---

[36] Schrumpf E, Charley H, "Texture of Broccoli and Carrots Cooked by Microwave Energy," *Journal of Food Science* 40 (1975): 1025–9.

[37] Lubec G, Wolf C, Bartosch B, "Aminoacid Isomerisation and Microwave Exposure," *Lancet*; 334, no. 8676 (Dec. 9, 1989): 1392–3, doi:10.1016/S0140-6736(89)91996-X.

[38] L. Petrucelli, GH Fisher, "D-Aspartate and D-Glutamate in Microwaved versus Conventionally Heated Milk," *Journal of the American College of Nutrition* 13, no. 2 (April 1994): 209–10.

was shown in a study published in *Food Additive and Contaminants*[39] in 1995 to release small amounts of BADGE into food during microwaving. Benzophenone is a component of ink on printed paperboard. This toxic chemical has been shown to migrate from the packaging into the food. PVC plastic films have been found to release plasticizers into the food when microwaved according to a study done in 1996.[40] We should never microwave plastics. Therefore, we should never heat plastic bottles for our babies. This is a serious health hazard that should be avoided. Use glass bottles, and heat them with water boiled on the stove or in a kettle.

---

[39] M. Sharman, CA Honeybone, SM Jickells, L. Castle, "Detection of Residues of the Epoxy Adhesive Component Bisphenol A Diglycidyl Ether (BADGE) in Microwave Susceptors and its Migration into Food," *Food Additives and Contaminants* 12, no. 6 (1995): 779–87.

[40] AB Badeka, MG Kontominas, "Effect of Microwave Heating on the Migration of Dioctyladipate and Acetyltributylcitrate Plasticizers from Food-Grade PVC and PVDC/PVC Films Into Olive Oil and Water," *Journal of Food Control and Research* 202, no. 4 (1996): 313–17.

CHAPTER 5

Supplements and Remedies

While breastfeeding provides baby with the healthiest start in life, some experts suggest supplementing since we live in a toxic world. Our healthy microbiome can easily be killed off, chemicals can enter our bodies through air, water, and food, and our food quality can be challenged due to inadequate minerals in our soils. In addition, there are a number of common ailments that can safely and effectively be treated with natural remedies, such as diaper rash, cradle cap, colic, gas, teething, and the common cold.

Supplements

Probiotics

A probiotic specifically formulated for infants will help lay a solid foundation for digestive health by fostering the growth of healthy bacteria. It also may help prevent allergic reactions such as eczema. I recommend beginning probiotics designed specifically for infants from day one of life.

Essential Fatty Acids

From as young as six months babies can be supplemented with essential fatty acids (EFAs). Essential fatty acids are fats that cannot be made in the body and must be obtained from food sources. This is an essential nutrient for brain and nervous system development and has been shown to support early vision system development in a large meta-analysis conducted by the Harvard School of Public Health.[41] I recommend nursing moms supplement with EFAs such as evening primrose oil, flax seed oil, or hemp in oil or capsule form. The EFAs will move through the breast milk to the infant. If your baby is on formula, I recommend adding approximately 2000 mg of EFAs to four cups of formula.

Vitamin C

Vitamin C is an excellent antioxidant that helps support healthy immune function. Vitamin C is needed for proper growth and development. It is also able to assist in moving toxins out of the body. Recommended dose for ages two and younger is 50 mg per day, which can be added to their bottle in liquid form.

Vitamin D

The best way to get our dose of natural vitamin D is from the sun, by exposing sunscreen-free skin to the sun for at least fifteen minutes per day. This can be through a window or taking your child for a walk outside every day. If your child is getting sun exposure on a daily basis, I don't recommend supplementing with vitamin D. I recommend supplementing with vitamin D if your child doesn't get adequate sun exposure (for example if you live in an area that tends to be overcast or during a really cold spell when going outside is difficult). Also, make sure to buy vitamin D3, which is the natural version. Vitamin D2 is often prescribed, and it's synthetic. Recent research is leading experts to recommend that all infants, including ones who are breastfed, be supplemented with vitamin D.[42, 43] This is to address an increasing prevalence in vitamin D

---

[41] JP SanGiovanni, S. Parra-Cabrera et al., "Meta-Analysis of Dietary Essential Fatty Acids and Long-Chain Polyunsaturated Fatty Acids as They Relate to Visual Resolution Acuity in Healthy Preterm Infants," *Pediatrics* 105, no. 6 (Jun. 2000): 1292–8.

[42] CL Wagner, FR Greer, "Prevention of Rickets and Vitamin D Deficiency in Infants, Children, and Adolescents," American Academy of Pediatrics Section on Breastfeeding; American Academy of Pediatrics Committee on Nutrition, *Pediatrics* 122 (2008): 1142.

[43] BW Hollis, CL Wagner, "Assessment of Dietary Vitamin D Requirements during Pregnancy and Lactation," *American Journal of Clinical Nutrition* 79 (2004): 717–26.

deficiency and rickets in infants in northern countries such as Canada. The recommended dose for infants is 200 IUs per day.

Zinc

Infants born prematurely and low birth-weight infants are at risk of zinc deficiency. Zinc is an important trace mineral that supports a healthy immune system, helping prevent respiratory infections and playing a role in proper reproductive organ growth and development. The recommended dose is 5 mg per day.

Multivitamin for Toddlers

I prefer that children get their nutrients from their foods, but the reality is that most toddlers are not achieving their nutritional needs for proper growth and development. A multivitamin that contains all the B vitamins, vitamins C, E, and A, as well as minerals including calcium, iron, zinc, magnesium, and selenium is a good way to ensure that their basic nutritional needs are being met.

Remedies for Common Ailments

Diaper Rash

Diaper rash is a red skin rash over any of the area in contact with the diaper. Typically, this occurs due to excessive moisture, diapers being too tight, sensitive skin, sensitivity to chemicals in diaper or in detergent, or a dietary irritant in baby's diet or in mom's diet of breastfed babies. Calendula cream can help soothe the skin, but the causative factors need to be addressed to have lasting results. Apply the calendula cream with every diaper change to the affected area.

Cradle Cap

Cradle cap is a crusty, flaking, plaque-like rash on baby's scalp. This can occur due to too vigorous and too frequent hair washing, or EFA (essential fatty acid) deficiency from not consuming enough EFAs through the diet. This can be treated naturally with coconut or sesame oil with a few drops of healing lavender essential oils added. Rub the oil mixture onto the scalp twice a day.

Colic

Colic is pain in the digestive tract, which, as medically defined, leads to sudden, inconsolable crying that lasts for three hours a day, occurs at least three days a week, and continues for at least three weeks. Common causes of colic include sensitivity to foods in mom's diet or in formula such as cow's dairy, caffeine-containing foods, wheat, corn, nuts, and spicy foods. A natural treatment for colic is external castor oil belly rubs. Massage castor oil onto stomach in a clockwise direction while baby is crying to help relieve pain. It is preventively helpful to do this daily before bedtime. For lasting results, food sensitivities need to be removed from the diet of the baby and/or mother.

Bloating, Burping, and Gas

Bloating, burping, and gas are all signs that food is not being effectively metabolized. Typical symptoms are a distended abdomen and releasing gas through burping or flatulence. This can be caused by sensitivity to foods in mom's diet or in formula such as dairy, caffeine-containing foods, wheat, corn, nuts, and spicy foods. A great natural remedy for this is the tissue salt Magnesia phosphorica 6x. Tissue salts are essential minerals that are needed for the function and health of the body and are gentle remedies that can be used safely with infants without any side effects. This product acts as a natural muscle relaxant. Take two pellets daily of tissue salt Magnesia phosphorica 6x.

Another tactic is gently pumping babies' knees into their chest, which helps move gas through the digestive tract. For lasting results, food sensitivities need to be removed from the diet of the baby or mother.

Teething

Signs of teething include drooling, runny nose with clear discharge, fever, looser stools, biting, sucking on fingers or pacifiers, or night waking (not sleeping through the night). Typically, this starts around five or six months and continues until they're about two and a half years old. Homeopathic medicines are gentle therapies that have been around for hundreds of years. They are dilutions of natural substances that work on the concept of "like curing like." This means that if a substance causes symptoms in a healthy person, it will cure similar symptoms in a sick person. The homeopathic Chamomilla 6CH can help soothe the symptoms of teething. In acute situations you can give two pellets of homeopathic Chamomilla up to every fifteen minutes. If you are worried about the infant choking on the pellets, you can dissolve the pellets in water and put drops of that water in the infant's mouth.

Common Cold

Some symptoms of the common cold include runny nose, cough, and sneezing. This occurs due to exposure to others with viral infections in combination with a weakened immune system. This can be treated with the botanical astragalus and/or echinacea to boost the immune system, along with vitamin C, zinc, and the homeopathic pulsatilla 6CH. Dose of astragalus and echinacea depends on the type and form used. Children can take about 250 mg of vitamin C and 10 mg of zinc. Take one pellet of homeopathic pulsatilla 6CH six times a day. It is okay to catch the common cold, but if colds last longer than seven days, and if you are catching colds more frequently than every three months, you have a weakened immune system, and the cause needs to be explored for causative factors.

Fevers

Fevers are actually a good thing. They are positive immune responses to an invading infection and are a sign of a healthy immune system. Fevers set up an environment that is not conducive for an infection to live. White blood cells that defend the body against invading infections work more effectively with an elevated body temperature. Infections do not survive in high temperatures. Fevers are a body's innate intelligence, so we should try to avoid fever reducers, which suppress the exact function that is helping the body to heal. If you reduce a fever, you confuse the immune system, whereby you do not fully recover from an infection, and this leads to an echo pattern where a child can be intermittently sick for a long period of time. We need to support the healing process even if it's uncomfortable. When we support the natural healing process, and the fever breaks on its own, we strengthen our natural immunity. The human body has an amazing ability to fight off infections and heal itself. We just need to harness its healing capacity. We can support the fever by applying cold packs to the child's neck. The homeopathic medicines aconite 6CH and belladonna 6CH help bring a fever down gently. You do want to watch the child carefully for danger signs of a fever: fever with temperatures over 104 degrees F, the child is confused, loses consciousness, starts to twitch, or seems hot on one side of the body and cold on the other.

Minor Cuts and Scrapes

When there is superficial bleeding or small skin wounds caused by stumbles or falls, these can be treated with tea tree oil, which has antimicrobial effects, and calendula cream, which soothes the skin. Dilute one or two drops of tea tree oil in a cup of water and gently dab the wound with the solution until the wound is clean, apply the calendula cream, and then apply a bandage.

Pain and Inflammation from Minor Injuries, Sprains, Strains, or Bruises

When a child gets a minor injury, the injured site will typically be red, swollen, and painful as the body mounts an inflammatory response to heal the underlying tissues. The natural remedies are not designed to stop the inflammation but to support and quicken the healing process. The homeopathic medicine Arnica montana 6cH can be helpful with treating minor injuries. Take two pellets of Arnica montana 6cH orally as often as every ten minutes as needed.

Insect Bites or Stings

Insect bites can get red and swollen at a well-demarcated area of the skin. This can occur from an insect such as a bee or wasp. Apis gel relieves itching and swelling. Apply gel to the affected area. Apis mellifica 6cH relieves the pain. Take two pellets orally as often as every ten minutes as needed.

Minor Sunburn

Sunburn occurs after exposure to the sun and the skin is red, swelling, and burning. This can occur with prolonged, unprotected exposure to sun. Aloe vera gel can heal and soothe the skin. Apply gel to skin as needed. The homeopathic Urtica urens 6cH can help with the burning pain. Take two pellets orally as often as every ten minutes as needed.

Common ailments	Natural Treatment	Instructions
diaper rash	calendula cream	Apply calendula cream with every diaper change to affected area.
cradle cap	coconut or sesame oil with a few drops of lavender essential oil	Rub oil onto scalp two times a day.
colic	castor oil externally	Massage castor oil onto stomach in a clockwise direction while they are crying to help relieve pain. It is preventively helpful to do this before bedtime.

Common ailments	Natural Treatment	Instructions
bloating, burping, and gas	tissue salt Magnesia phosphorica 6X	Gently pumping babies' knees into their chest helps move gas through the digestive tract. Take two pellets daily of tissue salt Magnesia phosphorica 6X.
teething	homeopathic Chamomilla 6cH	In acute situations can take two pellets of homeopathic Chamomilla 6cH up to every fifteen minutes.
common cold	astragalus, vitamin C, or homeopathic Pulsatilla 6cH	Dose of astragalus is dependent on the form it is consumed; refer to directions on the label. Take 250 mg of vitamin C per day. Take one pellet of homeopathic Pulsatilla 6cH six times a day.
minor cuts and scrapes	tea tree oil or calendula cream	Apply oil or cream to injury as needed.
pain and inflammation from minor injuries, sprains, strains, or bruises	homeopathic Arnica montana 6cH	Take two pellets of homeopathic Arnica montana 6cH orally as often as every ten minutes as needed.

Common ailments	Natural Treatment	Instructions
insect bite or sting	Apis gel relieves itching and swelling; homeopathic Apis mellifica 6cH relieves pain	Apply gel to affected area. Take two pellets of homeopathic Apis mellifica 6cH orally as often as every ten minutes as needed.
sunburn	aloe vera gel or homeopathic Urtica urens 6cH	Apply gel to skin as needed. Take two pellets of homeopathic Urtica urens 6cH orally as often as every ten minutes as needed.

CHAPTER 6

The Liver and Toxins

The Maturing Liver

The liver is one of the body's major detoxifying organs. The liver filters more than 1.4 liters of blood per minute. It removes bacteria, toxins, and any other unwanted substances from the blood circulation. This organ is constantly examining what comes into the body and deciding if it's useful or needs to be moved out of the body through very specific detoxification pathways.

The liver reaches full maturation at around four or five years of age. Even at full maturation a child's capacity to handle toxins is a lot lower than an adult, simply based on a pound-by-pound basis. Their systems are smaller, and their bodies are not fully developed, so this makes it challenging for them to handle large toxic loads. Their systems can be overloaded with toxins quickly and easily, so we need to be mindful of the amount our children are exposed to and work to reduce the load on their systems. An increased toxic load can affect the function of their body, and this can vary symptomatically from individual to individual (i.e., it can appear as eczema in one child, or asthma, or ADHD).

What Is a Toxin?

A toxin is anything our bodies do not recognize. Throughout evolution our bodies have been hardwired to recognize certain substances, which get broken down into smaller elements that are then used as our building blocks, including proteins, fats, carbohydrates, minerals, vitamins, and water. Anything other than these substances are seen as toxins by the body. Other substances that are viewed as toxins are foods that are not properly metabolized or broken down into smaller element building blocks.

Toxins in Our Food

Unfortunately, our food supply is infiltrated with a high toxic load including but not limited to pesticides, herbicides, insecticides, antibiotics, synthetic hormones, preservatives, food additives, and dyes.

Anytime we eat foods that contain substances our bodies do not recognize, it results in an increased load on our livers and a challenge to our bodies.

When we eat, our bodies break the food down into small components that are the building blocks of our bodies. We use them to make energy, repair tissues, and build cells. When we ingest substances that our bodies do not recognize, the substances get filtered out by the liver and then go through detoxification pathways, which essentially are packaging these unusable substances or toxins to safely move them out of the body (typically through the stools). Our bodies are hardwired to digest "real food." When we ingest foods that contain chemicals or are genetically modified or altered due to microwaving, heating, or chemical alternation processes, they are of no use to us. With an increased toxic load, the liver gets overworked and congested, like a clogged drain, making it difficult to effectively do its job. We need to feed our children foods that their bodies can recognize and turn into useful fuel.

Heavy Metals

The term heavy metal refers to the majority of metals, including lead, mercury, cadmium, and arsenic, that are five times heavier than water. In our modern world our environment, food, water, and the air we breathe expose us to these toxic metals, and with repeated exposure, these metals accumulate in our bodies. Heavy metal toxicity refers to an excessive buildup of heavy metals in the body. Heavy metals disrupt normal cell function, and these effects include

- Inflammation: Our bodies see these toxic metals as foreign substances and mount an inflammatory response to attempt to rid these toxic substances. When the toxic load is too high for the natural inflammatory mechanisms to move the toxic load out the of body, the body moves the metals out of circulation and into tissues as a protective mechanism. Metals in tissues will disrupt normal cell function.
- Nerve damage: Heavy metals have an affinity for the nervous system. Mercury toxicity has actually been shown to cause nerve degeneration. This can be exhibited as ADHD, autism, and learning disabilities.
- Kidney damage: Kidneys detoxify heavy metals and are susceptible to toxic metal-induced damage.
- Immune dysfunction: Heavy metals can disrupt our immune systems' ability to fight infections.
- Mineral disruption: Heavy metals bind to essential minerals and prevent proper function in the body.

The combined toxicity of numerous metals present in the body is much greater than the effect of each metal on its own. A study[44] demonstrated that a dose of mercury sufficient to kill 1 percent of tested rats, when combined with a dose of lead sufficient to kill less than 1 percent of rats, resulted in killing 100 percent of the rats tested.

Here are some potential sources of exposure:

Mercury

- Silver dental fillings are composed of 50 percent elemental mercury.
- Many vaccines contain thimerosal, a mercury-containing preservative.
- Dietary sources include large fish including tuna, swordfish, shark, and shellfish; and high fructose corn syrup.

---

[44] J. Schubert, EJ Riley, SA Tyler, "Combined Effects in Toxicity—Rapid Systematic Testing Procedure: Cadmium, Mercury, and Lead," *Journal of Toxicity and Environmental Health* 4, no. 5–6 (1978).

Lead

- Baby powder with talcum has been shown to be contaminated with lead.[45]
- Prior to the 1970s, lead was found in house paint, gasoline, and water pipes.
- Found in candle wicks, toys.

Arsenic

- insecticides, rodent poison, fungicides, drinking water, seafood, pressure-treated wood, rice

Cadmium

- cigarette smoke
- artist and automotive paint pigments, batteries (nickel-cadmium), and seafood

Aluminum

- antacids, antiperspirants, vaccines, baking powder, aluminum cookware, and cans

Environmental Toxins

In our everyday lives there can be exposures to environmental toxins that can enter our body and bloodstream and interfere in the proper function of the organs and the nervous system. Often, there are personal care products that claim that they are designed for babies or children, but are high in toxic chemicals. You must read labels and be cautious of substances that you put on your child, including creams, lotions, and

---

[45] G. Rehman, IH Bukhari et al., "Determination of Toxic Heavy Metals in Different Brands of Talcum Powder," *International Journal of Applied and Natural Sciences* 2, no. 2 (May 2013): 45–52.

powders, products you bathe your child in, and shampoos/conditioners you put in their hair.

We are exposed to many environmental toxins in our foods, our environment, and in our personal care products. They include

- plastics, especially microwaving foods in plastic containers; the plastics will seep into the foods;
- petroleum solvents in creams called petrolatum;
- preservatives in processed foods such as monosodium glutamate (MSG), sodium benzoate, nitrates, sodium nitrites, and ethylenediaminetetraacetic acid (EDTA);
- preservatives in personal care products such as parabens, sodium laureth sulfate, and diethanolamine(DEA);
- perfumes, fragrances, and dyes in body lotions and soaps;
- food coloring and dyes in foods; and
- any medications, including other-the-counter cough syrups and children's fever-reducers; these are synthetic substances that increase the toxic load on the liver.

Ways to Reduce a Child's Toxic Load

The best way to reduce our children's toxic load is to avoid their exposures orally and on their skin. Remember: anything you put on the skin gets absorbed into the bloodstream. Read all labels, and avoid putting chemical products on our children. Stick with pure, botanical-based products with no added preservatives. Let's feed our children "real" foods that their bodies will recognize and can help build the foundation of their health.

We can use gentle therapeutic drainage remedies that improve the function of the detoxification pathways to ensure that the toxic load is effectively moving out of the body. It is best to work with a licensed health care practitioner or naturopathic doctor to guide you on which remedies will be best for your child.

CHAPTER 7
The Developing Microbiome

The microbiome is the ecosystem of microbes, colonies of bacteria and fungi that live in our digestive tracts. Colonization of bacteria in the digestive tract begins early in life.[46] Early exposure comes from traveling through the birth canal and breast milk and is made up of much-needed nutrients and healthy bacteria.[47] The immune system requires early exposure to bacteria to mature properly.[48]

Researchers found that the gut microbial community differed markedly between the autism-like behavior group and the control group.[49] When studying children with eczema, it appears that reduced exposure to bacteria and changes in gut bacterial makeup from birth is the potential causative factor, as children with eczema lack bacterial diversity when compared to healthy counterparts.[50] Those individuals who developed celiac disease have a different bacterial microbe composition than healthy controls.[51]

The microbiome is essential for processing of nutrients, proper immune function and preventing disease progression. Diversity in this ecosystem is

---

[46] N. Elazab, A. Mendy et al., "Probiotic Administration in Early Life, Atopy, and Asthma: A Meta-Analysis of Clinical Trials," *Pediatrics* 132, no. 3 (2013): e666–76.

[47] C. Chassard, T. de Wouters, C. Lacroix, "Probiotics Tailored to the Infant: A Window of Opportunity," *Current Opinion in Biotechnology* (2014), 26C: 141–147.

[48] Ibid.

[49] JA Gilbert, R. Krajmalnik et al., "Toward Effective Probiotics for Autism and Other Neurodevelopmental Disorders," *Cell* 155, no. 7 (2013): 1446.

[50] E. Forno, A. Onderdonk, et al., "Diversity of the Gut Microbiota and Eczema in Early Life," *Clinical and Molecular Allergy* 22, no. 6 (2008): 11.

[51] N. Elazab, A. Mendy et al., "Probiotic Administration in Early Life, Atopy, and Asthma: A Meta-Analysis of Clinical Trials," *Pediatrics* 132, no. 3 (2013): e666–76.

critical for developing innate immunity and setting the stage for adaptive immunity that helps us distinguish self from non-self. It is a diverse microbiome with its twenty million genes that helps us resist disease.[52] Diversity in the microbiome can be a determining factor of our overall health and longevity.

We have acquired our own unique foundation of microbes in our digestive tracts that will affect our future health by age three. Researchers are discovering that gut microbes are involved in early brain development and affect neurology, possibly impacting cognition, emotions, and mental health.[53] These early years are a critical time for setting up the foundation for biological processes that will occur through childhood into adulthood.

Eating natural, fresh foods helps promote the growth of good bacteria,[54] and the fiber and nutrients in the foods help fertilize the healthy gut flora, hence the program outlined in this book will help to promote and support a healthy microbiome.

Threats to the Developing Microbiome

C-Section Deliveries

Our microbiome begins developing at the moment of birth. We get many microbes as we pass through the birth canal, so babies delivered by C-section miss gaining some key microbes from the birth canal[55,56,57,58], and this can be a contributing factor in future health issues.

---

[52] M. Blaser, *Missing Microbes* (Toronto: HarperCollins Publishers Ltd., 2014), 197.

[53] JA Gilbert, R. Krajmalnik et al., "Toward Effective Probiotics for Autism and Other Neurodevelopmental Disorders," *Cell* 155, no. 7 (2013): 1446.

[54] N. Elazab, A. Mendy et al., "Probiotic Administration in Early Life, Atopy, and Asthma: A Meta-Analysis of Clinical Trials," *Pediatrics* 132, no. 3 (2013): e666–76.

[55] Dominguez-Bello MG, Costello EK, Contreras M, Magris M, Hidalgo G, Fierer N, Knight R. "Delivery mode shapes the acquisition and structure of the initial microbiota across multiple body habitats in newborns." *Proceedings of the National Academy of Sciences* 107, no. 26 (2010 Jun 29):11971-5.

[56] Pender J, Thijs C, Vink C, Stelma FF, Snijders B, Kummeling I, van der Brandt PA, Stobberingh EE. "Factors influencing the composition of the intestinal microbiota in early infancy. *Pediatrics* 118, no. 2 (2006 Aug): 511-21.

[57] Biasucci G, Benenati B, Morelli L, Bessi E, Boehm G. Cesarean delivery may affect the early biodiversity of intestinal bacteria. *Journal of Nutrition* 138, no. 9 (2008 Sep):1796S-1800S.

Overuse of Antibiotics

We also need to be mindful of the overuse of antibiotics, as antibiotics kill off colonies of healthy microbes and decrease the diversity of the microbiome ecosystem. It is the diversity of the microbiome that can define how healthy we are in the future.

There is evidence that early life antibiotic exposures are increasing and worsening the risk of developing type 1 diabetes in terms of both the number of individuals affected and the age of onset.[59] Children who took antibiotics had more than triple the risk of developing Crohn's disease than those who were antibiotic-free.[60] A Canadian study showed double the risk of asthma in children who received antibiotics in the first year of life.[61]

Even short-term antibiotic treatments can lead to long-term shifts in the microbes colonizing our bodies.[62] Broad-spectrum antibiotics are capable of entirely wiping out rare microbes.[63] This can lead to loss of biodiversity, and even a small decline in biodiversity can make a community more susceptible to an introduced pathogen.[64]

Hand sanitizers and antibacterial soaps can kill off infectious agents, but as they make their way into your digestive tracts, they kill off the good, healthy microbes, similar to the way antibiotics do, so you do not want to use hand sanitizers or antibacterial soaps with your children. How does it get ingested? One example: we use the hand sanitizers/antibacterial soap and then touch or eat our food, and it makes its way into our digestive tracts.

---

[58] Biasucci G, Rubini M, Riboni S, Morelli L, Bessi E, Retetangos C. Mode of delivery affects the bacterial community in the newborn gut. *Early Human Development* 86 Supplement, no. 1 (2010 July): 13-15.

[59] M. Blaser, *Missing Microbes* (Toronto: HarperCollins Publishers Ltd., 2014), 171.

[60] Ibid., 178.

[61] Ibid.

[62] Ibid. 194.

[63] Ibid. 194.

[64] Ibid. 195.

Our Food

Livestock are given antibiotics, and then we consume the animal products. Even these trace amounts of antibiotics kill off good, healthy microbes in the digestive tract. Animals are meant to eat grass, not grains. When they eat the foods they are meant to eat, they have healthier gut flora. They absorb the proper nutrients such as healthy fats, which make grass-fed meats healthier and tastier. We want to consume organic (not injected with antibiotics or hormones), grass-fed animal proteins.

Our vegetables and fruits are sprayed with insecticides, pesticides, and herbicides that are designed to kill off bugs, but once we consume them, they also kill off healthy microbes in our digestive tracts and thus contribute to the decline in diversity in our microbiomes.

One of the most harmful broad-spectrum herbicides is glyphosate, the active ingredient in the commercially available herbicide Roundup. Glyphosate has been shown to disrupt the balance of gut bacteria; increase the ratio of pathogenic bacteria; damage the villi in the gut; impair cytochrome P450 enzymes, which play an important detoxification role in the body; and may be the cause of chronic diseases that are rooted in gut dysfunction.[65] There is an extremely strong correlation between of the use of glyphosate and increases in different diseases, including celiac disease, autism, type 1 diabetes, autoimmune disease, thyroid disease, kidney failure, and cancer.[66]

Environmental toxins, heavy metals, food additives and preservatives, and GMOs have been shown to disrupt the microbiome and can lead to potential health problems.

Poor diet, such as foods high in processed sugars, refined carbohydrates, and trans fats encourage growth of unhealthy bacterial overgrowths and throw off the microbiome balance.

---

[65] A. Samsel, S. Seneff, "Glyphosate, Pathways to Modern Diseases II: Celiac Sprue and Gluten Intolerance," *Interdisciplinary Toxicology* 6, no. 4 (Dec. 2013): 159–84.
[66] Ibid.

Our Water

Chlorine is a chemical that is added to our tap water to reduce or eliminate microorganisms such as bacteria and viruses. It is effective at reducing waterborne diseases. It is the most cost-effective way to disinfect our tap water, but not necessarily the safest or the best for long-term health.

Dr. Joseph Price, author of *Coronaries/Cholesterol/Chlorine* (1988), conducted a study[67] using chickens where one group was given water with chlorine and one without, and the groups were observed throughout their lifespan. The group raised with chlorine showed atherosclerosis in every bird, but the group without chlorine had no incidence of atherosclerosis. The author concluded that "it would be a common-sense conclusion that if regular chlorinated tap water is not good enough for the chickens, it probably is not good enough for us humans!"

Chlorine is an antimicrobial, meaning it kills living organisms. When we consume chlorine, it kills off our healthy bacterial terrain in our digestive tracts, leading to imbalance in our gut flora and disarming our immune system.

Chlorine reacts with organic matter that is naturally present in water, such as decaying leaves. This chemical reaction forms by-products called trihalomethanes (THMs) that are highly carcinogenic. The amount of THMs found in tap water depends on the season and where the source of the water is. Lab animals exposed to high levels of THMs have an increased risk of cancer. Several studies[68,69,70] on humans have found a link between long-term exposure to high levels of chlorination by-products and a higher risk of cancer. These pollutants can be odorless and tasteless but harmful to our health.

---

[67] Joseph M. Price, *Coronaries Cholesterol Chlorine* (Rogers, AR: Rhino Publishing SA, 2008).

[68] M. Panyakapo, S. Soontornchai, P. Paopuree, "Cancer Risk Assessment from Exposure to Trihalomethanes in Tap Water and Swimming Pool Water," *Journal of Environmental Sciences* 20, no. 3 (2008): 372–8.

[69] B. Tokmak, G. Capar, FB Dilek, U. Yetis, "Trihalomethanes and Associated Potential Cancer Risks in the Water Supply in Ankara, Turkey," *Environmental Research* 96, no. 3 (Nov. 2004): 345–52.

[70] TP Flaten, "Chlorination of Drinking Water and Cancer Incidence in Norway," *International Journal of Epidemiology* 21, no. 1 (1992): 6–15.

There is a link to breast cancer.[71,72,73] Women with breast cancer have significantly higher levels of organochlorines (chlorination by-products) in their breast tissue than women without breast cancer.[74] An epidemiological study[75] funded by Health Canada concluded that 14–16 percent of bladder cancers in Ontario may be attributed to drinking chlorinated water.

Chlorine is one of the easiest substances to remove from our water. It should be removed at point of use. Activated carbon filters can remove chlorine and its by-products. I recommend you not drink chlorinated water. Drink filtered water with chlorine and its by-products removed.

[71] DJ Hunter, SE Hankinson et al., "Plasma Organochlorine Levels and the Risk of Breast Cancer," *New England Journal of Medicine* (Oct. 30, 1997), 337: 1253–8.

[72] N. Kneger, MS Wolff et al., "Breast Cancer and Serum Organochlorines: A Prospective Study among White, Black, and Asian Woman," *Journal of the National Cancer Institute* 86, no. 8 (1994): 589–99.

[73] MS Wolff, PG Toniolo et al., "Blood Levels of Organochlorine Residues and Risk of Breast Cancer," *Journal of the National Cancer Institute* 85, no. 8 (1993): 648–52.

[74] C. Charlier, A. Albert, P. Herman et al., "Breast Cancer and Serum Organochlorine Residues," *Occupational and Environmental Medicine* (2003), 60: 348–51.

[75] WD King, LD Marrett, "Case-Control Study of Bladder Cancer and Chlorination Byproducts in Treated Water (Ontario, Canada)," *Cancer Causes and Control* 7, no. 6 (Nov. 1996): 596–604.

CHAPTER 8

Recipes

Homemade Formulas

Raw Goat/Sheep Milk Formula (birth to age 2)

4 cups of raw goat/sheep milk
1–2 mg B complex vitamin in liquid form
0.2 mg folic acid in liquid or powder form (goat's milk is deficient in this nutrient)
1/4 teaspoon flax seed oil
1 drop beta carotene (5000 IUs)
1 drop vitamin E (25 IUs)

Mix ingredients together and store in fridge until needed. Use glass bottles (first treated with boiling water to sterilize). Take note of the expiration date of the goat/sheep milk, as this will be how long the formula will last.

Rice Protein Formula (birth to age 2)

1 cup high-quality professional brand rice protein powder
8 cups filtered water
1/4 teaspoon sea salt
1–2 mg B complex vitamin
1/4 teaspoon flax seed oil
1 drop beta carotene (5000 IUs)
1 drop vitamin E (25 IUs)

Mix ingredients thoroughly together, and store in fridge in glass bottles (first treated with boiling water to sterilize).

Recipes to Begin at Six Months

Pureed Carrots

Steam 1 cup chopped carrots over 2 cups of boiling water. When carrots are soft, put carrots and 1/2 cup of the water in the blender until smooth in consistency. Serve immediately or freeze into ice-cube tray for future use.

Pureed Broccoli

Steam 1 cup of chopped broccoli over 2 cups of boiling water. When broccoli is soft, put broccoli and 1/2 cup of water in the blender until smooth in consistency. Serve immediately or freeze into ice-cube tray for future use.

Pureed Cauliflower

Steam 1 cup of chopped cauliflower over 2 cups of boiling water. When cauliflower is soft, put cauliflower and 1/2 cup water in the blender until smooth in consistency. Serve immediately or freeze into ice-cube tray for future use.

Pureed Zucchini

Steam 1 cup of chopped zucchini with skin over 2 cups of boiling water. When zucchini is soft, put zucchini and 1/2 cup of water in the blender until smooth in consistency. Serve immediately or freeze into ice-cube tray for future use.

Pureed Green Peas

Boil 1 cup of green peas in 2 cups of water. When green peas are soft, put green peas and 1/2 cup of water in the blender until smooth in consistency. Serve immediately or freeze into ice-cube tray for future use.

Mashed Yam

Peel yam and chop into smaller pieces. Boil yam in 2 cups of water. When yams are soft, pour water out of pot and mash yam until a smooth consistency. Serve immediately or freeze into ice-cube tray for future use.

Mashed Acorn Squash

Cut acorn squash in half with a very large knife directly through the center lengthwise. Scrape out the seed bulb, and lightly oil the open sides with organic extra virgin olive oil. Bake the two halves of squash on a baking sheet or shallow pan. Scrape the squash out of the baked skin into a mixing bowl. Mash the squash until it is a smooth consistency. Serve immediately or freeze into ice-cube tray for future use.

Mashed Sweet Potato

Peel sweet potato and chop into smaller pieces. Boil 1 cup of sweet potato in 2 cups of water. When sweet potatoes are soft, pour water out of pot and mash sweet potato until a smooth consistency. Serve immediately or freeze into ice-cube tray for future use.

Mashed Avocado

Remove skin and pit of avocado. Mash the fruit until it is a smooth consistency. Serve immediately.

Raw Cool Cucumber Soup

2 cups cucumber, chopped
1 cup zucchini, chopped
1 cup avocado, peeled and chopped
1 large lemon, juice
1 small garlic clove, minced
2 tablespoons cold-pressed olive oil
1/2 teaspoons salt
3 cups lukewarm filtered water

Blend all ingredients in a blender until smooth. Serve cold or at room temperature.

Recipes to Begin at Eight Months

Mashed Papaya

Cut papaya in half, spoon out seeds. Spoon out papaya, mash to a smooth consistency, and serve immediately.

Mashed Banana

Peel banana. Mash banana until a smooth consistency and serve immediately.

Apple Sauce

Peel and core 12 apples. Steam apples over boiling water. When apples are soft, put apples and 1/2 cup of water in the blender until smooth in consistency. Serve immediately or freeze into ice-cube tray for future use.

Pureed Peaches

Cut 6 peaches and remove the pit. Steam peaches over boiling water. When peaches are soft, put peaches and 1/2 cup of water in the blender until smooth in consistency. Serve immediately or freeze into ice-cube tray for future use.

Smoothie

Mix 1/2 cup of frozen berries with ice in a blender.

Recipes to Begin at Ten Months

Egg Yolks

Hard boil an organic egg. Remove the egg white, and serve the yolk. Egg whites have a protein in them called albumin that many infant's sensitive digestive tracts react with, therefore avoid egg whites until age two.

Puréed Meat

1/2 cup cooked meat (chicken, beef, etc.), cut into small pieces
1/4 cup water

In a food processor or blender, combine meat and water. Process for 1 to 2 minutes or until smooth. Serve immediately or freeze in an ice-cube tray for future use.

Beet Salad

Boil 1–2 beets in water until soft enough to poke a fork into them (can take up to 2 hours). Drain and cool, and then peel the skin off. Be careful, as beets can be staining. Cut into cubes. Enjoy hot or cold.

Cream of Carrot Soup with Leek and Fresh Ginger

Ingredients:
8 cups organic chicken, turkey, or vegetable stock
2–3 pounds carrots, peeled (use large mature carrots)

3 leeks (slice lengthwise, and wash out sand, using as much of the inner green leaves as possible, as it adds to the subtle flavor and adds a lot more fiber)

1 medium yam (peeled)

4 stalks celery

1 piece of fresh ginger root, peeled and grated, approximately 3 inches long (use a blender with the grater blade with about 1 cup of water. Strain and use immediately.)

1 teaspoon ground black pepper

1 teaspoon ground nutmeg

sea salt, to taste

Preparation:

In a large pot, bring stock to a boil.

Chop all vegetables into small pieces. (When the carrots are chopped into approximately 1/2-inch pieces, the next step is much easier than if you sliced the carrots into rounds.)

Sauté leeks, yams, celery, and carrots. Leeks, celery, and ginger are sautéed lightly until they are soft only. The real secret in the preparation of this recipe is in the browning (caramelizing) of the orange vegetables (carrots, yam, or squash). The browner (without burning) the better. This is the most tedious part of the preparation and may require several fry pans going at once. Caramelizing of the sugars in the mature carrots also distinguishes this dish's flavor from all the other carrot soup recipes.

Add the sautéed vegetables and nutmeg to the stock. Reduce the heat, cover with a lid, and simmer until the carrots and yams are soft. Be sure to use a temperature setting low enough to keep bottom from burning. Two hours should be sufficient.

Allow soup to cool to room temperature. Puree the soup in a blender in small batches, and add sea salt to taste. The soup should be thick and smooth. I have a large salad bowl that allows me to add all the cooled pureed soup before warming to serve or freeze for storage. This soup freezes very well. I am convinced it even improves the flavor.

To serve, reheat, but do not allow to boil.

Recipes to Begin at Twelve Months

Butternut Squash Soup

Ingredients:
2 tablespoons olive oil or sesame oil
2 onions, chopped
1–2 cloves garlic, finely chopped
1 tablespoon Jamaican-style curry powder or red curry paste
1 teaspoon ground coriander
6 cups chicken stock (homemade is best because you control the salt)
1 medium-sized butternut squash (about 3 pounds), peeled and cubed into
1- or 2-inch pieces
1/2 cup creamed goat's cheese
1/4 cup chopped parsley or cilantro

Preparation:
Squash may be difficult to peel. As an alternative, it can be cut in half with a very large knife directly through the center lengthwise. Scrape out the seed bulb and oil the open sides lightly with oil. Bake the two halves on a baking sheet facing up or shallow pan lined with foil. Scrape the squash out of the baked skin and set aside until ready to use. Squash can be prepared well ahead and frozen using this method or by peeling, cubing, and boiling.

In a large saucepan or Dutch oven, heat the oil to medium heat. Add the onions, stirring lightly for 2–3 minutes, and then add the minced garlic and sauté for an additional 2–3 minutes or until the onions are almost translucent.

Add the 1 teaspoon of coriander to the onions and garlic and sauté for another 2 minutes.

Add the chicken stock and the squash and bring to a boil. Add the curry powder, cover, and simmer the soup for about 30 minutes or until the squash is very tender. Stir occasionally.

Pour in batches into a blender or use a hand blender and blend until pureed. Return to saucepan, and add the cream cheese. Cook on low heat until the cheese is melted and the mixture is well blended, stirring frequently with a wire whisk.

Cajun (Stuffed or Mashed) Sweet Potatoes

Ingredients:
4 medium sweet potatoes
1/2 cup onions, finely chopped
1 tablespoon olive oil
1/2 cup celery, finely chopped
1 large tomato, finely diced
1/2 cup cooked raw spinach, finely chopped
1 tablespoon Cajun spice

Instructions:
Scrub potatoes and pat dry. Bake on cookie sheet for an hour at 400 degrees F.

Sauté onions in oil in frying pan. When soft, add celery. Reduce heat and steam until soft. Add tomatoes, spinach, and seasonings. Mix well.

When sweet potatoes are done, remove from oven.

They can be prepared either stuffed or mashed:

Stuffed—slice off the top quarter of the potatoes and remove pulp from shells. Place pulp in a bowl, blend well with Cajun filling, and stuff shells with mixture.

Mashed—remove pulp from sweet potatoes and mix with Cajun filling. Serve. (Skins may also be finely chopped into mixture.)

Serves 4 (stuffed) or 4–6 (mashed)

Coconut Chia Pudding

Ingredients:
2 cups unsweetened coconut milk
1/3 cup chia seeds
1/4 cup raw honey or local maple syrup
1/4 teaspoon cinnamon
coconut flakes and berries (for garnish)

Directions:

In a small bowl or large jar, stir together the coconut milk, chia seeds, honey or syrup, and cinnamon. Chill in the refrigerator for at least 4 hours or until the chia seeds puff and expand.

Before serving, stir once and spoon into serving dishes. Garnish with coconut flakes and/or berries and serve immediately.

Pudding may be stored in an airtight container in the refrigerator for up to 3 days.

Recipes to Begin at Eighteen Months

Crock-Pot Beef Chili

Ingredients:

2 pounds organic, grass-fed ground beef
1 onion, finely diced
3 cloves garlic, minced
2 (14.5-ounce) cans diced/whole tomatoes (organic, in water, no salt added, BPA-free cans)
4 stalks of celery, chopped
4 carrots, chopped
1 (15-ounce) can kidney beans (organic, in water, no salt added, BPA-free cans)
1 (15-ounce) can chickpeas (organic, in water no salt added, BPA-free cans)
1 (15-ounce) can pinto beans (organic, in water no salt added, BPA-free cans)
2 tablespoons chili powder
1 tablespoon ground cumin
1 tablespoon oregano
1 tablespoon parsley
1 tablespoon basil
1 tablespoon salt

Directions:

The night before, chop up the carrots, celery, onions, and garlic; put it all in a container; and stick it in the fridge overnight. Add all the spices to the container of vegetables.

Then brown the ground beef on the stove in a frying pan. When they cool, put then in another container and stick it in the fridge overnight.

In the morning, put all the ingredients into the Crock-Pot, turn the Crock-Pot on for 6 hours at low, and dinner is ready and warm when you get home in the evening.

Banana Fritters

Ingredients:
3 bananas, mashed
1 cup almond flour
1 cup goat's milk/almond milk
2 egg yolks, lightly beaten
1/2 teaspoon pure vanilla extract
2 tablespoons pure maple syrup
4 tablespoons olive oil

Directions:
Mix ingredients together in a mixing bowl.

Heat oil in medium pan over medium heat. Drop about 1 tablespoon of mixture into pan. Repeat and space out the fritters. Cook until golden brown (approximately 3 minutes per side). Flip fritter until other side is golden brown. Remove fritters from pan and place onto plate.

Creamy White Bean Veggie Dip

Ingredients:
1 can white cannelloni beans (organic, in water, no salt added, BPA-free can)
2 cloves garlic, minced
1/2 cup fresh dill
1/4 cup fresh lemon juice
1/4 cup olive oil
2 tablespoons almond yogurt

Instructions:
Blend all ingredients together in a food processor and serve chilled with vegetables of your choice. Refrigerate leftovers.

Strawberry Almond Yogurt Fruit Dip

Ingredients:
1 cup almond yogurt (available in most natural health food stores)
1 cup fresh strawberries
1 tablespoon raw honey

Directions:
Blend strawberries until pureed. Mix pureed strawberries, almond yogurt, and honey together. Best served chilled. Refrigerate leftovers.

Bean Salad

Ingredients:

Salad

2 to 3 cups green beans (fresh are best but frozen may be used in a pinch)
1 can six-bean blend (or use any bean you like: kidney, black, pinto, etc., organic, in water, no salt added, BPA-free cans)
1 can chickpeas (organic, in water, no salt added, BPA-free cans)
1 large sweet onion, diced
1 to 2 tablespoons fresh dill or to taste
3 tablespoons fresh chopped mint or 1 teaspoon of dried mint
1 to 2 tablespoons fresh chopped parsley

Dressing

1 teaspoon fresh chopped basil
1 tablespoon fresh chopped oregano
2 tablespoons balsamic vinegar
2 large cloves of garlic chopped or 3–4 small cloves of garlic
1 small onion coarsely chopped

2 tablespoons lemon juice
3 tablespoons olive oil
1 tablespoon prepared mustard (yellow, Dijon, or specialty, check for gluten-free)
1 tablespoon real maple syrup
salt and cracked black pepper to taste

Preparation:
Blend all dressing ingredients in a blender; adding mustard will create a creamy dressing that will not separate in oil and vinegar. Set aside. Add more olive oil to thin the dressing if required.

Drain and rinse canned beans in a sieve or colander to remove excess moisture.

Trim ends from fresh green beans and put into rapidly boiling water for approximately 2 minutes. Beans should be crisp. Submerge beans in ice cold water to cool quickly (stops cooking and retains color and crispness). Set aside to remove excess moisture, failing to remove moisture will result in a watered down flavor to the salad. Use paper towel if necessary

Cut green beans into 1-inch lengths. Combine the rinsed canned beans and other raw ingredients in a container that can be tightly sealed. Chop mint with a very sharp knife so as not to bruise and add to bean mixture. Add the dressing and toss to combine.

Allow salad to rest for 2 hours before serving. The salad will keep for several days in the refrigerator and improve in flavor.

Quinoa Salad

Ingredients:
1/4 cup quinoa
1 cup chopped celery
1 cup chopped cucumber
1/4 cup green onions
1/2 cup halved grape tomatoes
2 tablespoons olive oil
1 teaspoon pesto (homemade or store bought)
1/2 cup crumbled goat's cheese (feta)

Instructions:
Cook the quinoa according to directions on package. Mix all ingredients together and serve.

Rainbow Quinoa Salad

Ingredients:
1 cup tricolor quinoa
2 cups organic chicken stock
2 garlic cloves, minced
1/2 cup cucumber, chopped
1/2 cup celery, chopped
2 tablespoon parsley, chopped
1/4 cup grape tomatoes, halved
1/4 cup green onions, chopped
2 tablespoons olive oil
juice of 1 lemon
1/2 ripe avocado as garnish

Directions:
Cooked the tricolor quinoa in stock. Add all ingredients together. Garnish with sliced avocado.

Recipes to Begin at Twenty-Four Months

Zucchini Fritters

Ingredients:
2 medium zucchinis, grated with skin
10 sprigs of fresh flat-leaf parsley, finely chopped
2 large eggs, lightly beaten
1/2 cup almond flour
1 clove of garlic, minced
1 tablespoon of freshly grated lemon zest
sea salt to taste
4 tablespoons organic olive oil

Directions:

Combine zucchini, parsley, eggs, garlic, lemon zest, and sea salt in a medium bowl. Slowly stir in the flour.

Heat oil in medium pan over medium heat. Drop 1 heaping tablespoon of mixture into pan. Repeat and space out the fritters. Cook until golden brown (approximately 3 minutes per side). Flip fritter until other side is golden brown. Remove fritters from pan and place onto plate.

Banana Bread (Paleo, Gluten-Free, Sugar-Free)

Ingredients:
1/2 cup coconut flour
1/2 cup flaxseed meal
2–3 medium bananas
1/2 cup organic butter or coconut oil
1/2 cup chocolate chips
1/2 teaspoon cinnamon
3/4 teaspoon baking soda
1/2 cup raw honey
4 eggs
1/2 teaspoon vanilla extract
pinch sea salt

Instructions:

Preheat the oven to 350°F. Grease a 8½ × 4½–inch loaf pan with butter / coconut oil, or line the loaf pan with parchment paper.

Combine bananas, coconut flour, flaxseed meal, cinnamon, baking soda, salt, eggs, butter, vanilla extract, and honey in blender or food processor.

Pour mixture into a medium-sized bowl, and mix in the chocolate chips.

Spoon the batter into the loaf pan, and spread evenly with a spatula.

Place in the oven for 40–45 minutes or until a toothpick pierced in the center comes out clean.

Remove from oven and let it cool slightly (about a minute or so), and then carefully run a knife along the edges to make sure nothing is sticking. Carefully invert it onto a wire rack so that the bottom is lying flat. Let cool for 20–30 minutes before serving.

Asparagus Risotto

Ingredients:
5 cups chicken or vegetable stock
2 tablespoons extra virgin olive oil
1/4 cup unsalted butter, chopped, separated
1 onion, finely chopped
2 cloves garlic, crushed
1 1/2 cups Arborio rice
2 bunches (approximately 1 1/2 lbs) asparagus, trimmed, cut into 1-inch pieces
2 teaspoons finely grated lemon
2 tablespoons lemon juice, or to taste
1 cup grated goat's parmesan cheese or grated Manchego sheep's cheese

Preparation:
Bring stock to a boil in a saucepan over medium heat. Reduce heat to low, cover, and gently simmer.

Heat oil and half the butter in a large saucepan over medium heat. Add onion and garlic, cooking and stirring for 4–5 minutes or until onion is soft.

Add rice and cook, stirring for 2–4 minutes or until rice is hot and well coated in onion mixture. Do not let the rice brown.

Add 1 cup hot stock and stir continuously until stock has nearly all been absorbed. Add another cup of stock. Stir until stock has nearly been absorbed. Continue to add stock, a cupful at a time, stirring and allowing the stock to be absorbed before adding more.

Add asparagus to pan and continue to add stock, stirring frequently until mixture is creamy and rice is just tender (this should take about 20 minutes); add a little extra stock or water if necessary.

Add lemon rind, juice, remaining butter, and cheese to risotto. Stir to combine. Season to taste with salt and pepper. Serve immediately.

Notes: You may like to include chicken in this risotto. Cut cooked chicken thigh or breast fillets into 1-inch pieces. Add to risotto with the asparagus.

Gluten-Free Brazilian Cheese Bread

Ingredients:
1/2 cup olive oil or butter
1/3 cup water
1/3 cup goat's milk
1 teaspoon sea salt
2 cups tapioca flour
2 teaspoons garlic, minced
2/3 cup freshly grated goat's parmesan cheese or Manchego
2 beaten eggs (at room temperature for best result)

Directions:
Pour olive oil, water, milk, and salt into a large saucepan and cook over high heat. When the mixture comes to a boil, immediately remove from heat and stir in tapioca flour and garlic until it bonds. The mixture will be very thick and dry. Set aside to rest for 10 to 15 minutes.

Preheat oven to 375°F.

Stir the cheese and egg into the tapioca mixture until well combined, the mixture will be chunky like cottage cheese. Drop rounded, 1/4 cup-sized balls of the mixture onto an ungreased baking sheet (line with parchment paper for easy cleanup).

Bake in preheated oven until the tops are lightly browned, 15 to 20 minutes.

Chewy Chocolate Brownies (Gluten-Free)

Ingredients:
1 1/2 cups organic coconut palm sugar
1/2 cup butter
1/2 teaspoon salt
1 teaspoon pure vanilla extract
3/4 cup cocoa

3 large eggs
3/4 cup tapioca flour
1 teaspoon baking powder
1 cup semisweet chocolate chips

Directions:
Preheat the oven to 350°F.

Heat sugar, butter, and salt in a saucepan over medium heat. Constantly stir until the butter melts.

Pour mixture into a bowl, blending in vanilla and cocoa. Add eggs and mix well. Stir in baking powder, flour, and chocolate chips.

Pour batter into greased 8-inch square pan.

Bake for 33–38 minutes or until the top is set.

Let cool for 15 minutes before cutting.

Chocolate Cupcakes with Icing (gluten-free, dairy-free)

Ingredients:
2 medium eggs
3/4 cups raw honey
1 1/2 cups very finely grated zucchini
1 cup brown rice flour
1/2 cup organic cocoa powder
2 teaspoons baking powder
1/4 teaspoon sea salt

Directions:
Preheat the oven to 350°F. Grease the cupcake tray with coconut oil.

Separate egg yolks and egg whites into separate bowls

Mix the egg yolks and honey in a large mixing bowl. Beat in the grated zucchini followed by the flour, cocoa powder, baking powder, and salt. Beat again to make sure all the ingredients are well incorporated.

Beat the egg whites until white and fluffy. Gentle fold egg-white mixture into other mixing bowl.

Pour into cupcake baking cups and bake for 30 minutes.

Let cool completely before icing.

Icing

Ingredients:
3/4 cups honey
4 large egg whites
1/4 teaspoon sea salt
3/4 cup butter
1 teaspoon pure vanilla extract
1/2 cup of dark chocolate, melted

Directions:
Place honey, egg whites, sea salt, and butter in a big metal mixing bowl over a pan of boiling water. Stir with a clean metal spoon until all mixed together.

Then mix melted chocolate and vanilla into bowl.

Place in fridge to thicken.

Recipes to Begin at Three Years

Cucumber Maki Rolls (for people comfortable making sushi)

Ingredients: (makes 1 roll)
1 nori (dried seaweed sheets)
12 cucumber strips
1/2 cup of short-grain sushi-grade rice (calrose rice)

Directions
Rinse sushi rice. Cook 1/2 cup rice with 1 1/2 cups of water. Stir constantly.

Let sushi rice cool down.

Place nori sheet on bamboo rolling mat. Spread rice evenly over nori sheet. Place cucumber strips horizontally about 1/3 from edge. Roll nori sheet with a bamboo rolling mat.

Cut the roll into pieces with a sharp knife.

Rice Rolls

Ingredients:
1 rice paper wrap
shredded carrots, approximately 1/4cup
romaine lettuce, 1 large leaf, cleaned
vermicelli noodles (made from green beans and peas), handful (purchase at a natural health food store that has these specialty noodles)

Directions:
Place rice paper wrap onto flat surface. Cover with wet paper towel. Soak noodles for 10 minutes in warm water to soften them up. Boil noodles in water for approximately 2–3 minutes until noodles are soft, and then drain water and let noodles dry.

Remove wet towel from rice paper wrap—rice paper should be soft.

Place lettuce, carrots, and noodles in horizontal line slightly off-center on the rice paper. Roll, fold in edges, and continue rolling.

Rice Wraps

Ingredients:
red lentil and rice wrap (or rice wrap or spelt wrap)
1 tablespoon hummus
2 tablespoons beans
2 tablespoons peas
2 tablespoons corn
1/8 cup brown and wild rice
1 teaspoon Dijon mustard
1 tablespoon balsamic vinegar
1 teaspoon extra virgin olive oil

Directions:
Cook 1/8 cup brown and wild rice in 1/4 cup water. Add beans, peas, and corn.

Once cooked add extra virgin olive oil, Dijon mustard, and balsamic vinegar.

Lay wrap on flat surface. Spread hummus on one side of wrap.
Put rice, beans, peas, and corn in horizontal line slightly off-center.

Chocolate Pudding

Ingredients:
1 banana
1 avocado
1/3 cup coconut oil
1/2 cup cocoa powder

Directions:
Blend all ingredients together until smoothly combined.

Nut-Free Granola Bars

Ingredients:
1/2 cup pumpkin seeds, chopped
1/3 cup dried cranberries, chopped
1/3 cup sunflower seeds
1/3 cup sesame seeds
1/2 cup finely shredded unsweetened coconut
1/3 cup chia seeds
1/3 cup hemp hearts
1/3 cup of cacao nibs
1/3 cup of goji berries
2 eggs
1 teaspoon pure vanilla extract
1 tablespoon raw honey
1/2 cup dairy-free mini chocolate chips
pinch sea salt
pinch cinnamon

Instructions:
Grease a 9-inch square pan with coconut oil or line with parchment paper.
Preheat oven to 350°F.

Combine all the dry ingredients. Pour wet blend over dry and mix to fully combine. Pour into pan and press down evenly.

Sweet Potato and Banana Muffins

Ingredients:
1 large sweet potato
1 banana, peeled
3 eggs
2/3 cup flax seed meal
1/3 cup coconut oil, melted
1 teaspoon vanilla extract
1 teaspoon baking powder
1/2 teaspoon cinnamon
1/4 teaspoon baking soda
pinch salt

Instructions:
Preheat oven to 350°F. Cut sweet potato in half and place on baking sheet face up, and bake for 25–35 minutes until super soft. Remove skin.

Reduce oven temperature to 375°F.

Place soft sweet potato and banana in the blender or food processor and puree. Add flaxseed meal, baking soda, and baking powder, and cinnamon. Puree until completely broken down and smooth.

Then add the wet ingredients: coconut oil, eggs, maple syrup, and vanilla extract.

Puree until smooth.

Line muffin tin with paper or silicone liners and use spoon to pour ingredients into each cup.

Bake muffins for 25–30 minutes or until a toothpick inserted comes out clean.

Let muffins cool before consuming as it helps the muffins meld together a bit more.

Conclusion

We have the opportunity to make changes and truly give our children health advantage by focusing on feeding our children real, high-quality, nutritious foods that will properly nourish their bodies, feed their brains, and improve performance in all areas of their lives.

Our bodies are intelligent, and we need to honor that innate intelligence. Our bodies are able to convert the foods we eat into every cell, tissue, and organ that make up our body. Everything we eat literally nourishes every cell in our body. We need to give our children's bodies the proper building blocks to build a solid foundation of health. This involves feeding our children the right foods at the proper times in their developing lives. This is the best way to prevent disease and nurture health.

Since the beginning of human existence our bodies have been hardwired to digest "real" foods in their natural state. The further our foods are from being natural, the more difficult it is for our bodies to break them down and turn them into useful building blocks. If we want to build a healthy body, we need to avoid feeding our children processed, refined foods. (Refined foods are foods that are stripped of their nutritional value.) Often, refined foods are fortified with nutrients, which means the manufacturers have added back some of the nutrients to the processed food, but since it is not in its original, natural form, the bioavailability of the nutrients in greatly reduced.

We need to understand what "nonfoods" are. These are foods that may have caloric intake but have no nutritional value, so they serve no purpose in forming the foundation of the body. Examples of nonfoods are refined, processed sugars and flours, including candy, chocolate and chocolate bars, ice cream, pizza, hot dogs, and fast food. Children need to avoid or limit their consumption of nonfoods as these foods do not provide the body with any of the building blocks that contribute to forming a solid foundation of health.

The main building blocks of our body are proteins, carbohydrates, and fats. Proteins form the bones and muscles of our body. Carbohydrates are needed for creating the energy that feeds our cells. Fats form the cell membranes and the nervous system, including the brain. Healthy protein sources are meats, beans, nuts, and seeds. The healthiest complex carbohydrate sources include vegetables and fruits. Complex carbohydrates are rich in vitamins, minerals, and fiber, which are needed for the body to function optimally. Healthy fats such as avocado, fish, nuts, and seeds are important for proper growth and development.

Our bodies are made up of 75–80 percent water, so the liquid that fuels our bodies should be water, not juice or soda pop. Let's encourage our kids to drink clean, filtered water.

There is no doubt that we live in a fast-paced, over-scheduled society, where eating packaged, processed foods is far more convenient than preparing a fresh meal. But we need to get our priorities straight and realize that eating healthy foods is vitally important and should not be put on the back burner as a secondary priority. The best way to prevent chronic disease in adults is to start with feeding our children a healthy diet with real, fresh, natural foods and building a healthy body.

This is a diet plan for building a healthy human being. It will not only be beneficial for our children but for everyone in the family. Let's make health a priority for our children and give them an advantage in life.

APPENDIX A

Preconception Preparation

Giving our children the healthy advantage actually begins at preconception.

I understand this is not always possible, but if you are in the stages of planning to get pregnant, it is ideal that both the mother and father start preparing their bodies to be in the best health possible. I recommend this preconception preparation be about one year in length.

The first stage is that mother- and father-to-be should have an excellent diet. In addition to improving your health and the health of your unborn child, an excellent diet can help you have balanced hormones, and this will help with easier conception.

Diet is about 90 percent of getting into the best possible health. In the famous Pottenger cat study,[76] the diet that contained 100 percent raw milk and raw meat produced optimal health, where the cats had good bone structure, wide palates with plenty of space for teeth; shiny fur; reproductive ease; gentle disposition; and absence of parasites and disease. In comparison, the consumption of suboptimal nutrition of cooked meat or heat-processed milk resulted in physical deterioration; infestation of parasites; skin diseases; allergies; softening of bones; adverse personality changes; hypothyroidism; infertility; and degenerative disease. This deterioration got worse with each subsequent generation. When the parents changed their dietary intake to an optimal diet, the subsequent generation's health improved.

This study illustrates the problems of consuming a suboptimal diet on

---

[76] F. Pottenger, *Pottenger's Cats: A Study in Nutrition* (California: the Price-Pottenger Nutrition Foundation Inc., 2009).

our health as well as on the health of future generations, but it also illustrates that the huge implications of improving the parents' diet and health before conception can actually improve the health of the next generations. You have the opportunity to break the cycle of chronic degenerative disease and improve the health of future generations one child at a time.

Recommended Diet

Focus on

- a variety of low glycemic-index, nonstarchy vegetables and fruits
- wild fish, free-range chicken and turkey, grass-fed beef
- nuts and seeds
- nonwheat grains such as brown rice, quinoa, oats
- limited amount of natural sweeteners including maple syrup, honey, or stevia
- drinking a minimum of 6 to 8 glasses of spring, filtered, or reverse-osmosis filtered water
- herbal teas.

Avoid

- alcohol
- wheat
- cow's dairy
- pork
- refined sugars, especially high fructose corn syrup
- trans fats such as margarine, fried foods
- artificial preservatives such as MSG
- artificial sweeteners

Limit hypoallergenic foods:

- soy products except fermented
- peanuts
- corn

Here is a brief explanation as to why the soon-to-be mother and father need to avoid these particular foods.

Wheat and cow's dairy are inflammatory foods. They consist of large proteins that are difficult to break down, so these proteins sit in the digestive tract and lead to inflammation. Your body spends more energy trying to manage this inflammation and less energy on repairing and rebuilding other tissues in the body.

Alcohol, refined sugars, trans fats, and artificial preservatives increase the toxic load on the liver. Anything that is unnatural or a chemical is seen as foreign to the body. The liver is one of our major detoxifying organs, so when a foreign substance enters the body the liver has to put extra time and energy into packaging the substances and then attempting to move them out of the body, usually through the stools. Since the liver is responsible for more than five hundred processes in the body, it can often get overwhelmed. By decreasing these substances in your diet, you can decrease that toxic load and allow this organ to do its job a lot easier.

I have found that women who have optimally functioning livers do not experience nausea during pregnancy, whereas those who experience nausea have liver toxicity. The intensity of the nausea experienced during pregnancy correlates well with the degree of liver toxicity. In addition to feeling unwell during the pregnancy, the mother is also sharing her toxic load with her unborn child. If you don't want to experience nausea with pregnancy, spend some time preconception cleaning up your liver, as it is not a good time to clean up the liver during pregnancy or while breastfeeding due to the mobilization of toxins to the fetus or baby.

Pork or pig proteins are close to human tissue. This is why pig tissues are often used in human surgeries such as heart valves and prolapse repairs. Eating pork elicits an immune response in the body. What can happen over time if you continue to eat this food on a regular basis is you can instigate an autoimmune response in the body where the immune system has difficulty deciphering between self and nonself.

Supplements for Mother-to-Be

Folic Acid (1 mg/d)

The mother-to-be should be taking folic acid for approximately six months before she starts trying to conceive. Folic acid is utilized during rapid cell division and growth, as it is needed for the synthesis and repair of DNA. During days twenty-five to twenty-nine post conception in utero, neural tube defects can occur, and this is the point when many women still do not know they are pregnant. The lack of dietary folic acid is associated with birth defects such as neural tube defects and birth abnormalities such as cleft lip or heart defects in developing embryos. Taking folic-acid supplements can prevent these defects. Folic acid can be found in leafy green vegetables, beans, and meat.

Vitamin B6 (300 mg/d)

Vitamin B6, pyridoxine, affects the metabolism of estrogen and helps in estrogen utilization. I would suggest taking 300 mg per day beginning approximately six months before intended conception. Vitamin B6 levels are high in yams, leafy green vegetables, and legumes, so it would be beneficial to include these foods in your diet.

Other considerations

Movement

The body is designed to move. Movement increases blood flow, helps with lymphatic drainage, and improves digestion. Our lymphatic system is a secondary circulatory system that cleans up tissues and moves toxins out of the body. The lymphatic system does not have pumps and valves like the blood system to move the fluids through the body; instead, it depends on muscle activation to stimulate the movement of the fluid. Lymphatic drainage is stimulating the movement of the lymphatic system through muscle activation. Our ancestors moved as a mode of transportation; unfortunately, with urban sprawl, vehicles, and sedentary occupations our lifestyles lack movement. Therefore, we need to make an effort to schedule it into our lives. I recommend at least thirty minutes a day of any kind of movement such as walking, running, hiking, cycling, skiing, swimming, yoga, Pilates, tai chi, marital arts, or even cleaning the house or gardening.

Heavy Metals

Check heavy metal loads on the body. Heavy metals can be passed on to the unborn child in utero. Heavy metals affect nervous system function and development. If you can reduce your heavy metal load, you can decrease the transfer of heavy metals to your child. This can play a large role in giving him or her a healthy start to life.

The biggest heavy metal exposure is through dentistry. Ideally you want to safely remove metal amalgams from your mouth before pregnancy and go through a chelation program to remove the metals from your body so that you do not pass the heavy metal load to your child in utero.

The most effective way to check for heavy metal load is to do a provoked urine analysis. This involves injecting or ingesting a chelating agent either intravenously or orally. The chelating agent binds to metals, moves them into circulation, and then the kidney filters the metals out of the body. Following receiving the chelating agent, the individual collects their urine for six hours and then sends a sample to a specialized lab. The lab does an analysis for the physical presence of the heavy metals in the urine and sends out the results to the practitioner who has administered the test. This is the best way to evaluate the heavy metal load but will not be able to tell you what the total body burden is. A chelation program is a way to move metals safely out of the body. It needs to be designed by a licensed health care practitioner with specialized training in chelation therapy. The chelation programs depend on a number of factors including levels of heavy metals, which heavy metal levels are high, the state of kidney function, and the vitality of the person.

APPENDIX B

Pregnancy

We should aim to give our unborn children a head start. Mothers should ensure the best quality and quantity of food to meet their and the growing fetuses' needs. Remember that your unborn children will be taking all the nutrients they need in order to grow and develop properly. If you are already deficient in specific nutrients, vitamins, or minerals, they will not have the raw materials to properly build all the intricate systems of their bodies. If you only have enough to sustain your health, you will soon become deficient as your little fetuses, over the next nine months, take what they need to grow. I recommend taking supplements in addition to following a complete, healthy diet.

An infant can become sensitive to a food that the mother eats during pregnancy. I recommend pregnant mothers avoid hypoallergenic foods including wheat, cow's dairy, pork, soy, peanuts, and refined sugar. Try to eat organically grown foods. This reduces the toxic load being passed to your fetus.

Recommended Diet

General Guidelines

Focus on

- a variety of low glycemic-index, nonstarchy vegetables and fruits;
- wild fish, free-range skinless chicken and turkey, grass-fed beef;
- nuts and seeds;

- limited amount of natural sweeteners, including real maple syrup, raw honey, or pure stevia;
- drinking a minimum of six to six glasses of spring, filtered, or reverse-osmosis water; and
- herbal teas.

Avoid

- alcohol
- wheat
- cow's dairy
- pork
- soy products except fermented
- peanuts
- refined sugar
- sweeteners such as artificial sweeteners, high fructose corn syrup
- trans fats such as margarine, fried foods
- artificial preservatives such as MSG, processed foods
- coffee and all caffeinated teas

Supplements for Pregnant Woman

Multivitamin

A high-quality prenatal multivitamin ensures all the important nutrients for both mom and baby are met. The multivitamin should include vitamins A, C, D, E, K; iron; zinc; bioflavonoids; CoQ_{10}; and choline.

Vitamin A intake should not exceed 6,000 IUs per day from all sources; too much can be toxic and has been known to cause birth defects. Recommended dose is 5000 IUs per day.

Vitamin C plays a vital role in forming connective tissue, cartilage, bones, nerves, and healthy gums and teeth, and in preventing infections. Recommended dose is 1000 mg per day.

Vitamin D is needed for the development of good teeth and strong bones. Increasingly, research is revealing the importance of vitamin D in protecting against a host of health problems, including bone pain and muscle weakness, and increased risk of death from cardiovascular disease, cognitive impairment, severe asthma in children, and cancer. Recommended dose is 1000 IUs per day. Much higher levels are safe and may be needed by some people. Check with your clinician for a safe amount to take.

Vitamin E deficiency during pregnancy can lead to low-weight infants and childhood asthma. Recommended dose is 10 mg per day.

Vitamin K may reduce the risk of intraventricular hemorrhage (IVH), bleeding into the fluid-filled spaces in the brain that occurs most often in premature infants.

Iron is needed to maintain adequate iron stores in the mother. Too little iron in the mother may result in anemia, which has been associated with low birth-weight babies, premature birth, and maternal mortality. Recommended dose is 30 mg per day.

Zinc is required for proper fetal growth and immunity. Recommended dose is 15 mg per day.

Bioflavonoids may reduce risk of miscarriages. Recommended dose 40 mg per day.

CoQ_{10} may prevent spontaneous abortions (the body self-aborting) and is essential for health of all human tissues and organs. Recommended dose is 4 mg per day.

Choline (lecithin) is an important precursor for neurotransmitters, the building block that is critical for nerve and brain development in an baby and part of every cell membrane in the body. Increasing choline in the mother can increase choline content in the breast milk. Recommended dose is 40 mg per day.

B Complex

A B complex vitamin is important during pregnancy, especially for the folic acid content needed to prevent neural tube defects. Thiamin (B_1), riboflavin (B_2), and niacin (B_3) have been shown to contribute to higher birth weight in infants. Pyridoxine (B_6) can help relieve morning sickness and nausea. Cobalamin (B_{12}) is needed for the normal function of the brain and nervous system and assists in blood formation. Recommended dosages: folic acid, 1000 mcg per day; thiamin, 1.5 mg per day; riboflavin,

1.6 mg per day; niacin, 17 mg per day; pyridoxine, 2.2 mg per day; and cobalamin (B_{12}), 2.2 mcg per day.

Calcium-Magnesium

To help prevent hypertensive disorders of pregnancy, such as preeclampsia, and to help ease leg cramps and improve baby's health, a calcium–magnesium supplement can be helpful. Recommended dosages: calcium, 600 mg per day; magnesium, 300 mg per day.

Essential Fatty Acids (EFAs)

EFAs are important for preventing pregnancy-induced hypertension and for balancing hormones, regulating bowel movements, and supplying the essential building blocks for the offspring's brain and nerve development. Recommended dose of omega-3 fatty acids from vegetable sources (e.g., flax oil, hemp oil, evening primrose oil) is 2000 mg per day, which is about the equivalent to eating an avocado.

Probiotics

To maintain a healthy digestive system throughout pregnancy, and to ensure proper absorption of dietary nutrients that help both mother and baby maintain optimum health, probiotics should be an essential part of daily supplement intake. Recommended doses: Lactobacillus acidophilus, 1 billion CFUs (colony forming units); Lactobacillus casei, 1 billion CFUs; Bifidobacterium infantis, 1 billion CFUs.

Gingerroot

Several studies have shown that ginger can alleviate nausea and vomiting during pregnancy. Fresh gingerroot can be used in cooking or prepared as a tea; ginger is also available in extracts, tinctures, capsules, and oils.

Other Considerations

Environmental Toxins

Any substance that goes on the skin or scalp gets absorbed into the bloodstream, so be cautious when selecting shampoos, conditioners, soaps, lotions, creams, laundry detergents, hair dyes, and makeup. Read through the ingredients and try to stay away from chemicals such as parabens and EDTA (an acid widely used to dissolve lime scale), which are common preservatives, as well as known carcinogens, cancer-causing agents when absorbed through the skin.

APPENDIX C

Vaccinations

This is an extremely controversial topic and a very important decision you'll need to make for your child's health and future. The majority of parents make this decision blindly, simply "go with the flow," and follow what their pediatrician suggests. Parents need to make an informed decision and understand the pros and cons of vaccinations.

The truth is there are risks involved in getting vaccinations and risks involved in not getting them. We commonly only hear one side of the story (pro-vaccines). It is important to understand both sides so that you can make an informed decision. The long-term effects of vaccines have yet to be effectively researched.

There is evidence of a correlation between vaccinations and increased susceptibility to allergies[77] and inflammatory bowel disorders.[78] Allergies are often found in cases of inflammatory bowel disease (IBS) as the irritated lining of the bowel mucosa allows for greater entrance of infectious agents into the bloodstream, increasing allergic and inflammatory responses throughout the body.

---

[77] TM McKeever, SA Lewis, C. Smith, R. Hubbard, "Vaccination and Allergic Disease: A Birth Cohort Study," *American Journal of Public Health* 94, no. 6 (June 2004): 985–9.
[78] NP Thompson, SM Montgomery, RE Pounder, AJ Wakefield, "Is Measles Vaccination a Risk Factor for Inflammatory Bowel Disease?" *Lancet* 345, no. 8957 (Apr. 29, 1995): 1071–4.

The Immune System

The immune system begins to develop in utero and continues to meet new challenges throughout our lives, reaching full maturation around seven years of age. The immune system's function is to maintain clear boundaries between what is allowed into our bodies and what needs to be removed. Our immune system protects us against invading microorganisms, including bacteria, viruses, fungi, and parasites.

We have two types of immunity: nonspecific and specific. We are born with a nonspecific immunity that provides us with a general response against a wide variety of foreign invaders. This consists of physical barriers that protect our body, skin, and mucous membranes.

The specific immunity includes a memory of previously encountered organisms, so if the body comes across that organism again, it is able to recognize and identify it and develop specific immune responses that allow the body to rapidly and directly respond to this infection.

When the body is exposed to an infectious agent such as a virus or bacteria, the immune system is activated. White blood cells go to the area to attack the infectious agent. The lymphatic system moves the unwanted microorganism to the lymph nodes, where white blood cells, called lymphocytes, produce antibodies to the infectious agent. Macrophages digest and destroy the infectious agent. Lymphocytes called B cells mature in the bone marrow and produce antibodies that bind to specific infectious agent. Then a B memory cell is produced, which stimulates immunity in the future against the same particular infectious agent. Each B-lymphocyte is a highly complex cell with approximately one hundred thousand immunoglobulins on its surface that identify only specific infectious agent. Different immunoglobulins (Ig) have specialized functions within the body. IgA is found in the mucous membranes to protect against invading microorganisms. IgG is the main antibody for bacteria and viruses and is involved in stimulating immunity in the baby even prior to birth. IgM is formed in the initial stages of most immune reactions. Other lymphocytes spread throughout the body through the blood, to the lymph, and go to the thymus gland, where they become T cells. T cells recognize the difference between invading cells, substances that need to be removed from the body, and cells that are allowed into the body.

An example of specific immunity is when a person contracts and recovers from an infection such as mumps, chicken pox, or measles; then they have lifelong immunity to that specific infection.

Vaccines work on the principle of activating our specific immunity. Injecting a small amount of an antigen or infectious agent into the body will trigger an initial immune response, and a second injection of the vaccine will enhance the reaction and further the antibody formations, creating a specific memory of that organism. Future exposure to the organism should then allow the body to quickly recognize and mount a full-scale response against the organism.

In natural infections, most infectious agents enter the body through the respiratory system or digestive tract (mucous membranes). This stimulates the IgA response, followed by the IgG and IgM antibodies. Most vaccines enter the body through an injection into the bloodstream. Therefore, most vaccines bypass the IgA response. Vaccinations attempt to bypass natural immune-system pathways in an attempt to acquire unnatural immunity. Vaccines do not establish the same type of immunity that natural exposure to a disease does.

Immunity is rarely induced after one vaccination, thereby necessitating numerous shots to stimulate the full antibody response, and boosters are often needed when antibody responses begin to diminish. Unfortunately, vaccine adverse-reaction incidence frequently increases with increasing numbers of injections.

Vaccine Ingredients

A major concern regarding vaccinations is the safety of vaccine ingredients. Very little research has been done on the long-term effects of the chemical agents used in vaccines.

- Aluminum is added to vaccines in order to increase the immune response so that a lesser amount of the active ingredient and fewer doses are used. Aluminum is a neurotoxin, a heavy metal that can be toxic to the human nervous system.
- Formaldehyde is used in vaccines to reduce the toxicity of microbial toxins. Formaldehyde is a known carcinogen.

- The presence of thimerosal, a mercury derivative, in some vaccines is used to prevent the contamination of vaccines with bacteria and fungi. Mercury is a toxic heavy metal.

Children are ten times more susceptible than adults to toxic effects of chemicals. Children are less capable of eliminating toxins due to their immature organ systems.

When toxins are injected into infants as part of vaccines, they can interfere with the normal development of the immune system, resulting in an increased susceptibility to infections and chronic immune disorders.

Blood-Brain Barrier

The blood-brain barrier is a selective barrier that lets very few substances come in contact with the brain and nervous system. This is an innate protective system that protects our nervous system from damage.

The blood-brain barrier in an infant is not fully developed until about twelve months of age. Therefore, the brains of fetuses and infants are at an increased risk of neurotoxins, including the common vaccine ingredient aluminum. Aluminum has the potential to interfere with neurotransmitters such as glutamate, which are essential for normal brain development. Aluminum has the potential to cause persistent inflammation in the brain. These are huge potential risks in vaccinating a child before complete development of the blood-brain barrier.

Perspectives on Vaccinations

Some people's perspective on the focus of preventing childhood disease is so important that the occasional severe adverse effects are considered necessary casualties or sacrifices for the greater benefit of humankind. Common reactions such as fever, screaming, appetite loss, and swelling and inflammation are considered minor side effects.

You as a parent need to weigh the risks associated with your child contracting specific childhood diseases in comparison to the risk associated with your child getting the vaccinations. Unfortunately, it becomes the concept of playing statistical roulette with your child's life.

We are told that vaccines are responsible for the decline of polio and smallpox, but the reality is that infectious diseases were already on the decline before vaccines were introduced. After World War II the incidence of infectious disease started dropping on its own due to better sanitation, such as clean water, central heating, and a higher-quality food supply. Better sanitation means infectious disease does not spread as easily.

On a regular vaccination schedule, infants receive twenty-eight doses of ten different vaccines by age two. Injections of multiple vaccines may overburden the infants' immature systems. The recommended vaccination schedule begins with four injections that include a total of sixteen different strains of viruses and bacteria. This means an infant's immune system is challenged to respond to sixteen different antigens simultaneously at two months of age. It is definitely rare for an infant to naturally be exposed to numerous diseases and chemical challenges all at once.

It is important to realize you have choices. You can choose to follow the regular vaccination schedule, you can choose to opt out of certain vaccines, you can choose to delay vaccines to when the child is older and his or her immune system is more mature, or you can choose to not vaccinate your child at all. I recommend reading books specifically dedicated to this topic and become informed before you make this crucial decision for your child.

Recommended Readings

Romm, Aviva Jill. *Vaccinations: A Thoughtful Parent's Guide: How to Make Safe, Sensible Decisions about the Risks, Benefits, and Alternatives.* Rochester, VT: Healing Arts Press, 2001.

Bailetti, Katia, ND. *Childhood Vaccinations: Answers to Your Questions,* 2nd edition. Toronto: Inhabit Media, 2010.

Diodati, Catherine JM. *Immunization: History, Ethics, Law, and Health.* Windsor, Ontario, CA: Integral Aspects Inc., 1999.

Index

About the Author

Dr. Melina Roberts is a licensed naturopathic doctor. She graduated from the University of Waterloo with an honors bachelor of science degree in kinesiology. She has her doctorate of naturopathic medicine from the Canadian College of Naturopathic Medicine in Toronto. In addition to her studies, she has pursued specialized training with leaders in the field of medicine, learning about medicine, natural healing, and effective testing and therapies in different parts of the world. She has more than eleven years of clinical experience. She has come to understand that if we can begin to change the health of our pediatric population, we can improve the health of our human population.

Dr. Roberts is the founder of the Advanced Naturopathic Medical Centre in Calgary, Alberta, Canada's comprehensive center for biological medicine, where she has a busy, successful private practice. She is passionate about health and enjoys sharing her knowledge. She happily resides in Calgary, Alberta, with her husband and daughter and enjoys skiing in the mountains.

TRUE DIRECTIONS
An affiliate of Tarcher Perigee

OUR MISSION

Tarcher Perigee's mission has always been to publish
books that contain great ideas. Why? Because:

GREAT LIVES BEGIN WITH GREAT IDEAS

At Tarcher Perigee, we recognize that many talented authors, speakers,
educators, and thought-leaders share this mission and deserve to be published –
many more than Tarcher Perigee can reasonably publish ourselves. True
Directions is ideal for authors and books that increase awareness, raise
consciousness, and inspire others to live their ideals and passions.

Like Tarcher Perigee, True Directions books are designed to do three things:
inspire, inform, and motivate.

Thus, True Directions is an ideal way for these important voices to
bring their messages of hope, healing, and help to the world.

Every book published by True Directions– whether it is non-fiction, memoir,
novel, poetry or children's book – continues Tarcher Perigee's mission to publish
works that bring positive change in the world. We invite you to join our mission.

For more information, see the True Directions website:

www.iUniverse.com/TrueDirections/SignUp

Be a part of Tarcher Perigee's community to bring positive change in this
world! See exclusive author videos, discover new and exciting books, learn
about upcoming events, connect with author blogs and websites, and more!
www.tarcherbooks.com

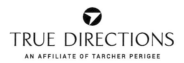

TRUE DIRECTIONS
AN AFFILIATE OF TARCHER PERIGEE

Printed in the United States
By Bookmasters